I, MICROBIOME

A Secret To Healthy And Balanced Human Body

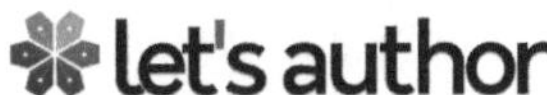

ADVANCE PRAISE

"The hottest potatoes in the microbiome world are tackled by "Therapy Takes up a Notch with Microbiomes." If you look at what laypeople are posting on social media these days about microbial transplantation or phage therapy, it's clear why this chapter is a must-read. The authors take a lot into consideration: What do we know about a particular microbial community and a specific disease? How to manipulate microbiota safely? Additional aspects like pharmacomicrobiomics, genetic background, hormonal status, individual microbiome composition (affected by drugs or affecting drug efficacy, toxicity), and personalization make this chapter so valuable."

—Rudi Schmidt, EVP Precision Medicine Asklepios Hospitals,
Managing Director Broermann Research,
CEO !mmunetrue, Germany

"A highly welcome and authoritative review of the state of the field today. Our knowledge of the microbiome is growing so rapidly, that this extensively researched and comprehensive book is the perfect foundation for scholars and entrepreneurs alike."

—Dr. Sven Sewitz, Director of Biodata Innovation,
Eagle Genomics, UK

Vladimir Jakovljevic

Debojyoti Dhar,

Edda Russo,

Amedeo Amedei,

Aruna Rajan,

Nina Vinot,

Ashok K. Sharma,

Manuela Pausan,

Alan Marsh,

Kristin Neumann,

Marco Pignatti,

Sofia Popov

First Printing: 2022

Hardcover ISBN: 978-81-952590-8-3
Paperback: 978-81-952590-7-6
Ebook: 978-81-952590-3-8

Illustrations by Veer Misra
All Illustrations are for representational purpose only.
Typeset by Manoj Gupta
Edited by Jyotirmoy Chaudhuri
Print by Saurabh Printers

Disclaimer: While every effort has been made to assure the accuracy of the information contained in this book, it is not intended as a substitute for medical consultation with a physician. The publisher and the authors are in no way liable for the use of the information contained in this book.

LetsAuthor
www.letsauthor.com

To my wife, Ivona.

— Dr Vladimir Jakovljevic

TABLE OF CONTENTS

PREFACE

THE word 'microbiome' is heard often these days. In the 1980s, during my primary school years, genetic engineering was a magical word one could hear in the newspapers and on television as back then we had no internet. After I got bored with common subjects such as math and physics in my school, I decided to study molecular biology and learn about genetic engineering. It didn´t take long before I realized the vast complexity of living organisms, cells, genes, structures, and processes, many of which we still don't know much about. At some point I thought that my chances of understanding the basic principles of life were higher with simpler organisms (or as simple as possible in biology) and so I shifted my focus to microbes—organisms typically made of only one cell. I became fascinated with all the possibilities microbes and microbial biotechnology had to offer such as helping us to diagnose, cure or prevent a disease, improve our food or everyday products, clean the environmental damages we make, and so on. During the next decades, I studied how microbes cause diseases, how they move, how they sense chemical and physical signals, etc.

About ten years ago, I learned about the next generation of DNA-sequencing technologies and the concept of microbiomes. I quickly realized the huge possibilities these new technologies will bring. The leap was as big as when we discovered the microscope or telescope. It instantly allowed us to see so unimaginable things. Since then, I carefully and passionately followed the developments in the field.

The word 'microbiome' has become a buzzword in the media. A buzzword spreads quickly and soon appears on all the web platforms and little devices we carry in our bags and pockets. But remember when we played Chinese whispers or "deaf telephones" as kids, often the last person never would get the initial word right. Unfortunately, the same is happening with scientific discoveries nowadays. Many internet gurus and conspiracy theoreticians get a lot of media space. Most scientific topics become a source of fun or heated debates on social media to the extent that someone's health gets affected by misinterpretation of the knowledge. With something as trendy as the microbiome, there will be certainly a number of people who will see this as an opportunity for earning, self-promotion, or both. Many will claim they can, for example, look into your microbiome and, just as they do by looking into a crystal ball, they can tell you what to eat, what to drink, or how to live your life healthily. This is as much real as looking into the crystal ball.

This is why a book on human microbiomes that skips the "deaf telephones" and brings the scientific truth in the most direct manner to awakened readers is the need of our times.

There are already several good books about human microbiomes on the market. However, these mostly cover a specific topic such as gut microbiome, nutrition, a particular health condition, or a specific set of health conditions. A few of them though have touched on several topics which will be also discussed further in our book. To our best knowledge, our book will be the first one trying to cover all aspects of human microbiome science and its applications as broadly as possible. However, the field is developing so rapidly that probably an update for some chapters will be needed in a couple of years and we are aware of that.

Finally, while we thought about an appropriate title for the book, the story of a robot from the cult book (and later also a movie) *I, Robot* by the famous science-fiction author Isaac Asimov, came to our minds. It has a symbolic connection to microbiomes because, during the past many millions of years on planet Earth, they evolved to live in a symbiotic relationship with humans and other living creatures. They have no intention to hurt us and, if we treat them right, they can serve us well too.

[Disclaimer: This book doesn't provide any therpeutical or medical advice.]

I hope you enjoy the book.

—Vladimir Jakovljevic, PhD
In Heidelberg, 3 May 2022

ACKNOWLEDGMENTS

THIS work would not be possible without the LetsAuthor open authoring platform and its stellar team. They first connected with me with the idea to write a book about human microbiomes. For that I am deeply grateful to Dr. Saumita Banerjee, the founder of Lets-Author, Namarita Kathait, the book manager, and all the members of the LetsAuthor team, for long and fruitful discussions, organizing meetings with co-authors, solving technical issues, their patience, and all the creative work and the ideas they brought in.

I am grateful to Dr. Manuela Pausan, Dr. Debojyoti Dhar, Dr. Ashok Kumar Sharma, Dr. Edda Russo, Prof. Amedeo Amedei, Nina Vignot, Aruna Rajan, Sofia Popov, Dr. Kristin Neumann, Alan Marsh, and Marco Pignatti for accepting invitations to be co-authors of the book, for their time, support with crowdfunding, their patience, and all the great ideas and contributions.

I would also like to thank all people who helped in the creation of the book by financially supporting our crowdfunding campaign, disseminating the preorder campaign information, giving critical feedback, or supporting us in other ways.

Special thanks go to Vuk-Dimitrije Velickovic, Natasa Moravic-Balkanski, Andreas Adam, Simone Giesler, Dr. Darja Wagner, Dr. Ferenz Paldy, and all the others who directly or indirectly helped the establishment of my company Microbiome Power, without which my visibility to the outside world and therefore, the initiation of this book would not be possible.

My endless gratitude goes to my family for their unconditional love and patience during all the moments I have not spent with them while working on the book.

Finally, I thank all my teachers and mentors, since my undergraduate studies, during my Ph.D. studies, and during my postdoctoral research, who helped me to learn and to grow my passion for microbiology and microbiomes.

—Dr. Vladimir Jakovljevic

INTRODUCTION

OFTEN thought of as the "aha" or eureka moments in the history of humankind, there have always been discoveries marking a turning point in eras. While there is no written evidence about the discoveries of fire, wheel, metal melting, and so on, we do know about one aha moment that happened in 1674 AD when Antonie van Leeuwenhoek saw living microorganisms under his microscope. It took another two centuries before the works of Louis Pasteur, Robert Koch, and other scientists gradually convinced people that diseases don't originate from "bad air" spontaneously—out of nothing—or by any other mysterious causes.

Cut to the twentieth century. While it was marked by two world wars and nuclear weapons, it brought us informatics and genetic technologies. We learned that a molecule called DNA is responsible for a human to be called a human, microbe a microbe, and tulip a tulip. Thanks to these and other technological advances, during the last twenty years we witnessed the birth of new machines able to read billions of A_T_C_G letters of DNA-written code in a matter of hours and the price of a few dollars. People named them "Next Generation Sequencing (NGS)," to be distinguished from the "old" DNA-sequencing technologies.

To describe these microbial communities better, scientists coined the term "microbiome"—a "collection of all microbial genetic material in a given environment." In the scientific literature, we also find the term "microbiota"— a "collection of all microorganisms in an environment." These two terms are used interchangeably. However, it is important to remember that microbiome is a broader term. As we will see ahead in the book, there might be many microbes that are yet to be discovered.

We learned that microbes cause diseases. Recently, however, we started to realize that changes in our microbial communities can have a tremendous influence on our health and well-being. Just as the millions of species that exist on Earth each contribute to the delicate balance that enables and sustains life on this planet, the microbiomes of our body, along with our cells and organs, contribute toward maintaining a healthy, functioning body and mind. This surely makes one wonder in a philosophical sense—what is "me" after all?

With the advances in microbiome research, it also became clear that we need to revise our definition of disease-causing microorganisms, also known as pathogens. Many of them are normal microbial residents in and on our bodies. Only if the conditions rapidly change and a microbial community shifts from a balanced state to an imbalanced one, a particular microbe (or microbes) in the community can become dominant, causing the disease.

The book traverses from our current knowledge about different human microbiomes, through available methods for microbiome analysis and the efforts researchers and entrepreneurs are making to use this knowledge for new disease diagnostics, therapy, and improvement of our general well-being. As the Indian-American entrepreneur, Naveen Jain has said, we hope that by using microbiome-based technology, soon we will reach a state where human disease will be only a matter of choice, not bad luck.

PART I

HOW IT ALL STARTED: OVERVIEW OF HUMAN MICROBIOMES

CHAPTER 1

IT'S NOT ONLY THE GUT

"Once upon a time in a garage, somewhere in California..."

This is how probably most future scientific tales will begin.

IN truth, something similar happened somewhere between 1994 and 1998 in several "garages" around the world to the new DNA-sequencing technologies, commonly called Next Generation Sequencing, or shortly NGS. This shift in technology is illustrated by a massive increase in sequencing costs of the first human genome (the complete genetic material of a human) from $2.7 billion[1] to $600,[2] as priced nowadays.

Soon after the NGS capabilities became obvious, the Human Microbiome Project (HMP), aimed at characterizing microbial communities of the various parts of the human body and their role in health and disease, was launched in the United States.[3] Since then, an explosion of other studies and projects arose, on various human microbiomes worldwide, with thousands of publications and dozens of entrepreneurs stepping into this new field.

As a result, our understanding of the composition, diversity, functions, and evolution of human microbiomes tremendously increased. However, it is still far from complete. Many of the popular literature, news articles, and blogs only address the human gut microbiome.

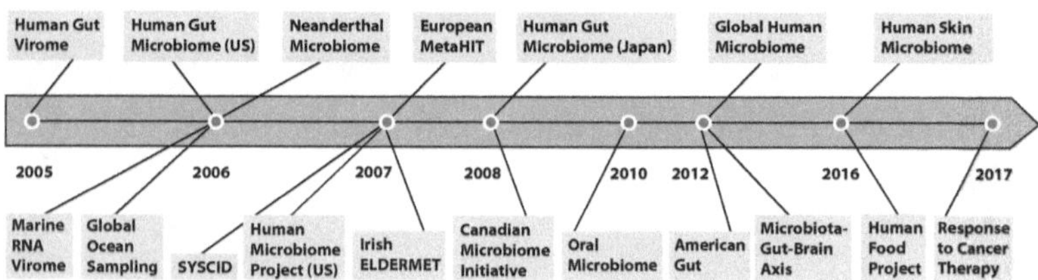

Fig. 1.1   Timeline of important projects in microbiome research.

Source: Adapted from Arogyam Analytics of the Microbiome Whitepaper

In this book, you will find that it's not only about the gut. The topic is much broader. To begin with, we will shortly introduce the most important microbiomes present at different human body sites.

Skin: A Favorable Environment

Skin is our first barrier to the outside world, with a surface area of about 1.5–2 square meters (m^2) on average. If we consider all micro-appendages on it, then the skin surface estimates go up to $25m^2$.[4] It's thus not particularly surprising that such a large surface is covered with microbes. As a warm and humid environment with the availability of essential minerals and nutrients, it is a great habitat for many different kinds of microorganisms. Typical inhabitants of our skin are bacteria, viruses, and fungi—not to frighten the germaphobes—, and also some small microscopic animals such as mites. Most of these organisms have been characterized and cultivated, but there are others whose existence is acknowledged only from sequencing (NGS) data. Estimates are that there are at least 600 different microbial species on our skin.[5]

Just as different parts of a big meadow might be covered with different plants, depending on its exposure to the sun, rain, or wind, so are different "hills and valleys" of our skin covered with different microbes. For example, distinct kinds of bacteria are found around sites near the glands producing our skin's grease (sebum), other kinds in the warmer and humid areas of armpits, and others in the colder or

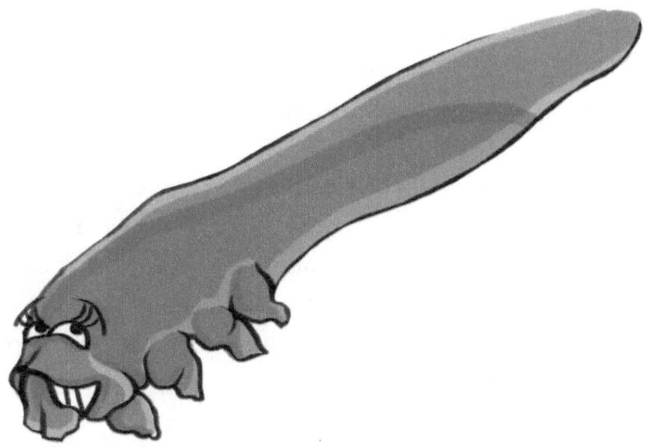

Fig. 1.2 *Demodex folliculorum*, a typical resident of human skin

dry sites such as fingers and toes. Even the two palms of our left and right hand have different microbial communities.[6]

Furthermore, there is variability between the skin microbiomes of men and women, different ethnicities, and people with different lifestyles or from different climates.[7] How we treat our skin is equally important: excess use of antibiotics, disinfectants, shampoos, soaps, detergents, and cosmetics, all can cause large variations in the composition of our skin microbes. As we age, the structure and chemical composition of our skin—and therefore skin microbiomes—change too.

Lively Community of Oral and Respiratory Microbiomes

The human oral cavity is a warm and humid place through which we inhale and exhale around 22,000 times a day and where everything we eat or drink goes through. So, it may not come as a surprise that there are a lot of microbes in there. Estimates are of around 700 different species, each with a preference for a different region: some like to dwell around our teeth, some prefer gums, others our cheeks, tongue, or palate. These local teams of microbes can greatly differ between two different persons, depending on their lifestyle, the food they consume, or their age.[8]

Till recently, people have believed that our lungs are more or less free of microbes unless we suffer from a disease of the lungs. We now know that's not true. Although the number of microbes is decreasing as we go down our airways, this small community seems to be very lively and diverse, and, as we will discuss later, it may have a profound influence on our health and immunity.[9]

Stomach and Gut Microbiome: The Most Heavily Researched

Microbes were the first colonizers of our planet, which a few billions of years ago was not so green and blue, but rather a hot soup, unfriendly to the kind of life we know today. During the dawn of life on Earth, microbes evolved to live in places such as rocks, under huge pressures at the bottom of the oceans, near hot springs and volcanos, or under the ice. One example of these so-called "extremophile" microbes is *Helicobacter pylori*, a bacterium happily swimming at the pH value of 1–1.5, in effect in acid solution strong enough to melt metal.[10] Our stomach is therefore exactly a place where it can thrive, and as we will see later, it may play a role in our health.

If we travel further down our gastrointestinal tract, we come to the small intestine where the stomach acid is neutralized and half-processed food is available. Again, a good environment for microorganisms to thrive. Unfortunately, because our methods for sampling the content of the small intestine from living humans are still not very advanced, our knowledge about the microbiomes living down there is lower in comparison to the ones in our mouth or the colon.

Finally, the last part of the journey of the gastrointestinal tract is through our large gut or colon. This is a real haven for microbes, given that the remainder of food stays here relatively longer, due to favorable

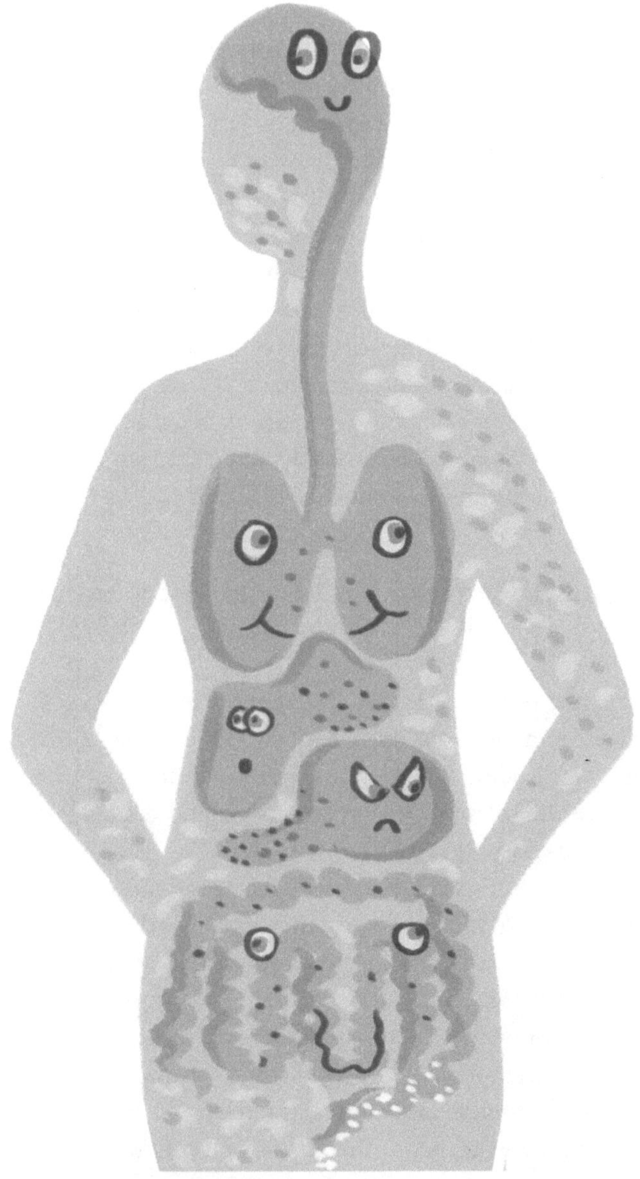

Fig. 1.3 Various microbiomes are present all-over human body (estimated number of species in brackets): skin (>600); oral, nasal and respiratory (>700); gut (500-1500); urogenital (>100)

temperature and humidity. This is also the part of the gut that we know the most about and is currently a large topic of research in the human microbiome field, with samples from here easily obtained out of stool or fecal material. Estimates vary from 500 to over 1,500 various microbial species in our gut, which may differ due to our age, nutrition, and our physiology.[11,12] As we will see further throughout the book, the gut is not only important for the final absorption of the nutrients and liquids from the food, but also for the proper development and functioning of our immune system and our brain, thereby affecting our whole body. Researchers and entrepreneurs worldwide are heavily engaged in this area and we are learning new things about the microcosmos in our gut on an almost daily basis. By the time this book is out, there will be probably new lessons to learn about the influence of the gut microbiome on our health and well-being.

Significance of Urogenital Microbiome

Similar to the respiratory tract, the upper urinary tract and bladder (as well as brain, placenta, and breast) were once considered a sterile environment. Today, this view has changed, and researchers have investigated the roles of these microbiomes and their significance in health and disease.[13]

The microbiome of the male genitals (penis and testis) and their role in male reproductive health and sexually transmitted diseases (STDs), has been largely neglected until recently.[14] For this reason, we must admit that our knowledge about the human reproductive microbiome comes mostly from the studies of the female genital tract.

The female reproductive microbiome, with more than 50 different microbial species on average, has relatively lower diversity in comparison, for instance, to the gut or oral microbiome. However, it shows diversity between different parts of the female reproductive tract: from the vagina to the cervix and uterus. Despite the influences of the hormones (e.g. menstrual cycle, pregnancy, or lifestyle) and differences among human subpopulations (e.g. Indo-European and African women), the vaginal microbiome represents a relatively stable community.[15,16] There is an evolutionary reason for this: the vaginal microbiome is not only important for female health, but also successful reproduction, immunity, and healthy microbiomes of the offspring. The vaginal microbiome may, in this sense, be the most beautiful example of the mutually harmonious relationship between our species and the microbial world.

With an increase in our knowledge about human microbiomes, we are constantly learning new things about the diversity of the microbiomes of different human body parts. However, this is just scratching the surface. In the following chapters, we will explain how the whole process of discovery of new microbial species, their functions, and interactions with the human body occurs. Further, we will provide an overview of the current applications of the knowledge about human microbiomes in therapy and beyond.

PART II

HOW ARE THEY ANALYZED: TOOLS AND TECHNIQUES

CHAPTER 2

SAMPLING AND STORING MICROBIOMES

IMAGINE a couple of Westerners somewhere in the savannah of Tanzania trying to get verbal consent from the local hunter-gatherer tribal people to sample their poop. You might think it is a recording of the next BBC documentary about indigenous people of Africa or another Hollywood comedy. However, this is only one example of what microbiome researchers have to go through if they want to compare gut microbiomes between different human populations.[1]

To study human microbiome samples, the first step is to isolate them from their natural environment. Methods for sampling generally depend on the body part from which they are isolated. For example, stool samples are relatively easy to collect while microbiomes of other parts such as human lungs or urogenital organs could be more challenging.

Understanding the Sampling Methods

Skin samples are typically obtained by cotton swabs or tape strips, although other methods such as scrapping or biopsy are sometimes used.[2] The mouth is relatively easy to sample, either by collecting saliva, swabs, mouthwashes, or by scraping dental plaque.[3] The stomach is more difficult to reach but thanks to the advancements in endoscopic techniques, it is nowadays much less risky for a gastroenterologist than a few decades ago. Distal small intestine is more difficult to sample but the pill-like robotic devices, which can travel through the intestine and collect microbes along the way, are a great innovation for sampling intestinal microbiomes.[4]

Collection of stool is the most frequently used method of sampling human gut microbiomes, in particular the large intestine and colon. Different technical solutions for stool collection have been developed, from pocket-sized swab kits for home use, to completely automated systems.[5]

Vaginal samples are typically collected using sterile swabs, spatulas, or brushes which are sold as kits, similar to those used for gut or oral microbiomes.[6] Usually, vaginal sampling is performed by a gynecologist but in some cases, it can be done at home. Microbiomes of the other parts of the female reproductive tract, such as the cervix or uterus (womb) can be sampled only at a specialist clinic. The same is valid for the other "hard to reach" microbiome samples, such as lung, bladder, blood, eye, or even human brain. These are all done by a specialist using special instruments or techniques which should definitely not be tried at home.

Why Safe Storing of the Microbiome Samples is Important

After microbiome samples are collected, they usually need to be transported to the laboratory where the analysis is performed. This is where the next difficulty arises. The laboratory can be just around the corner or it can be thousands of kilometers away. Depending on the intended applications, storage protocols can be very different.

If the next step is DNA sequencing, keeping microbial cells alive is not important, only preserving DNA. Fortunately for all living beings on our planet, DNA is a relatively stable molecule. It is usually enough to keep it in the stabilizing chemical solution (a buffer) and not expose it to extremely high temperatures.

Further, we know that DNA "letters" are transcribed into the other "letters" of a molecule called RNA, which then finally provides information about the protein that'll be made in the cell. Instead of extracting DNA from the cell, we can extract RNA. The problem with RNA, however, is that it is lesser stable molecule than DNA and tends to break down within minutes. To preserve RNA intact, it can be frozen within seconds (so-called "quick-freeze") by soaking it in liquid nitrogen and kept deep-frozen (at -80°C) until use. Similarly, stability of the proteins from the microbiome samples (e.g. stool) at room temperature is troublesome, and quick,deep freezing is the best option. Since deep freezing is not easily available in a home setting, the alternative is to store in special stabilizing buffers[7] and keep samples cooled when possible.

If living microbes are needed for a therapy such as Microbiome Transplantation (explained in Chapter 12) preservation of the viability and the original diversity of the microbial communities is crucial. The typical way of storing living bacteria for longer periods is quick/deep freezing using special media or freeze-drying (lyophilization). There are currently several biobanks in the world (such as OpenBiome in the US, Asia Microbiota Bank in Hong Kong, BiomeBank in Australia, Leiden University in the Netherlands, and several other clinics in Europe) in which stool samples of healthy donors are tested, processed and stored for potential further use in microbial therapy.[8]

If we want to study living microbes, we need to cultivate them in the laboratory. In the next chapter, we will explain some of the basic techniques to grow microbes and provide examples of how the interaction between microbe and the host can be studied.

GROWING MICROBES AND HOST-MICROBE MODELS

Louis Pasteur, the father of modern microbiology, came up with the idea to support microbial growth by providing bacteria with some homemade soup. In his experiment, he observed the growth of microbes on certain types of food. The liquid nutrient media for growing bacteria to this date is called "boullion," meaning "broth" in French.[1] Gradually, Pasteur's original homemade recipe got upgraded to more precisely defined mixtures of liquids and various growth formats, and the simple "Erlenmeyer" glass flasks got replaced by plastic multi-well plates and instruments for the cultivation of hundreds of samples simultaneously.

Another level of microbial cultivation came also from a soup, though, this time the traditional Japanese seaweed soup called *Tokoroten*. The legend says people observed that during long cold winter nights *Tokoroten* became solid, jelly-like. The seaweed jelly soon became very popular in the southeastern Asian kitchen, especially for preparing sweets, and by the mid-nineteenth century, as sea trading routes from Europe to South-East Asia became more active, it was introduced to the continent and named agar-agar (from the local Malay name for the red algae from which it is derived). Another legend says that one summer day in 1882, a girl named Fanny, who worked

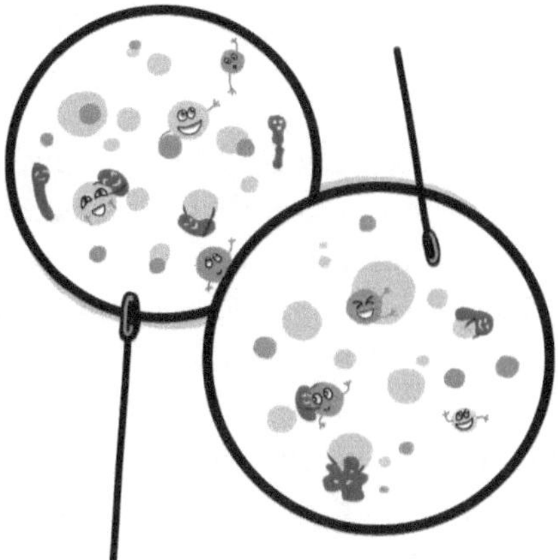

Fig. 3.1   Petri-dish, a plate covered with
agar-agar jelly is still used as a standard
to cultivate microbes in the laboratory.

as a technician in the laboratory of the famous German microbiologist Robert Koch, got advised by her Dutch neighbor (who had lived in Indonesia for a long time) to add some agar-agar in her pudding. She was delighted that the pudding didn't melt in the warm weather and got the idea to try to use it for the growth of Koch's microbes in the lab. Another colleague in his lab named Julius Richard Petri used agar-agar-based media in the culture dish, and this is how the famous "Petri-dish" was born, and is still used in microbiology laboratories all around the world. By the time both liquid and agar-agar-based media were developed to grow and select only special microorganisms of interest.[2]

The sad news is that with all of our present soups, gels, and other methods, we can grow only a tiny fraction of all microorganisms present on our planet. It is estimated to be less than 1 percent. The remaining 99 percent or more are sometimes called "microbial dark matter."[3] As we will see further, even our most powerful methods and computational predictions from the assemblies of microbial DNA sequences can give us a certain probability of finding new but uncultivable, microbial species.

Models to Study Host-Microbe Interaction

Beyond the ability to grow microbes, the next level of analysis is to test them in a situation closer to real life. The Latin term "*in vitro*" (literally, "in glass") is often used to describe experiments in a test tube, without a living model organism. In the meantime, *in vitro* has been broadened to various kinds of laboratory equipment, materials, and techniques. For instance, scientists have developed systems to simulate the gut environment and analyze natural specimens of microbes, such as stool samples. Sometimes these systems are simpler, simulating only one gut compartment (e.g. colon), while more advanced systems have several compartments, simulating conditions even of the complete human gastrointestinal tract.[4]

Another way to study how the host responds to a microbiome or how the host and microbiome mutually interact is through cell lines. The cervical cancer cells of Henrietta Lacks (known by many researchers around the world as "HeLa" cells), became a crucial part of history as the first cells possible to propagate endlessly in the laboratory. Since then, many cell lines were isolated from other organs (unfortunately, mostly from cancer cells), such as the small and large intestines. These cell lines are often used to study the interaction between the microbes and the host (human) cells, not only as a culture in a dish but also in more advanced systems such as Organoids, Transwell System, and Gut-on-a-Chip.[5]

The next level of studies falls somewhere between *in vitro* and on living animals (*in vivo*). These are called "*ex vivo*" methods, describing a situation where tissue or an organ, for example, a part of a human or animal gut, is physically removed from an organism for examination in a special chamber. These systems are used to measure the transport of drugs or other substances through the gut barrier. More advanced systems of this type also allow experimenting on many multiple samples simultaneously, in the so-called "high-throughput" format.[6]

> "Apparently, there was only one other species that was smarter than the dolphins, and they spent a lot of their time in behavioral research laboratories running around inside wheels and conducting frighteningly elegant and subtle experiments on man. The fact that once again man completely misinterpreted this relationship was entirely according to these creatures' plans."
>
> —Douglas Adams, *Hitchhiker's Guide to the Galaxy*

Modern biomedical sciences would be very difficult to imagine without experiments on laboratory animals such as rodents. A big breakthrough and an enabler for modern microbiome science was the discovery of the so-called "germ-free" (GF), "gnotobiotic", or "microbiome-free" rodent models (mostly mice and rats), which are animals born and raised in a completely sterile environment. Another approach to creating similar GF animals is through antibiotic treatment, drastically reducing all or eliminating selected bacteria. Using these animals, scientists can compare the effects of defined microbes or microbial mixtures on dietary habits, changes in animal behavior, etc. GF mice are expensive to raise and maintain and, due to their severe malfunctions in different organ systems, some experiments may not be possible to perform. Antibiotic treatment is a cheaper and relatively easier option, though its main deficiency is that it may not completely eliminate all bacteria.[7]

Other animal models for microbiome studies include zebrafish, fruit flies, and a roundworm called *Caenorhabditis elegans*. All of them are easier to cultivate under GF conditions and on a larger scale than the rodents. Indeed, zebrafish have some similarities to the human endocrine and nerve system.[8]

As for other human drugs, each microbiome-based drug candidate needs to successfully withstand standardized clinical trials to get licensed. Clinical trials are typically conducted by so-called Clinical Research Organizations (CROs). Some CROs are specialized in conducting trials for human microbiome therapies and probably more of them will appear in the years to come.

CHAPTER 4

TOOLS FOR ANALYSIS OF MICROBIOMES

Sequencing

It took more than twenty years since the discovery of DNA as hereditary material of all living beings and determination of its chemical structure, before techniques for the routine "reading" of the genetic code (namely A, T, C, and G "letters" of DNA), also known as DNA sequencing, became available. The complete overview and history of all DNA-sequencing technologies (many of which are not in use anymore) go far beyond the scope of this book. In short, until the late 1990s, the "old" DNA-sequencing methods were able to "read" only a few hundreds of the ATCG "letters" at once, and with maximally few dozens of samples simultaneously running on one sequencing machine (aka "DNA sequencer").

In 1998, after the Human Genome Project was completed (with costs reaching $2.7 billion) it became clear that new sequencing methods and instruments with the ability to process many samples simultaneously (aka "high-throughput") and at lower cost were needed. So, several groups of researchers independently started to develop several such methods, nowadays known as "Next Generation Sequencing" or "NGS." As mentioned in Chapter 1, the NGS methods have been fueling microbiome research from the very beginning.

Which are the Leading NGS Technologies?

On 9 September 2021, David Klenerman and Shankar Balasubramanian were awarded the 2022 Breakthrough Prize in Life Sciences—the world's largest science prize.[1] This was in recognition of their discovery of the first method for massive parallel DNA-sequencing, also known as Sequencing by Synthesis (SBS). In this method, DNA is broken into thousands of small pieces which are then immobilized on the surface of a chip, multiplied many times, and each copy decoded by incorporation of fluorescently labeled DNA "letters" A, T, C, or G. Signals are detected by excitation of the fluorescent dies by a laser and read by super-sensitive digital cameras. Solexa, the company which David and Shankar established in 1998 was bought in 2007 by Illumina, currently the biggest sequencing provider globally. Latest generation instruments from Illumina (NovaSeq 6000) produce up to 6Tb of data, meaning up to 40 billion of short DNA reads (each between 150-250 "letters" long) in a single sequencing run (13-44h). This high-throughput allows each single DNA "letter" of a genome to be repeatedly sequenced (read) many times, which is often expressed by the terms "sequencing depth" or "X-fold genome coverage." For example, NovaSeq can sequence 48 human genomes at 30-fold coverage in less than two days.[2] This means every A, T, C, or G in each of the 48 human genomes is read 30 times, greatly increasing the "reading" accuracy. Using this method, bacterial genomes which are 200 to over twenty thousand times smaller than the human genome can be sequenced with even higher precision (high depth) or with many more genomes simultaneously.

Ion Torrent/Ion Proton sequencing is another NGS platform owned by Thermo Fisher corporation. Instead of fluorescently-modified "letters" and optics, Ion Torrent uses hydrogen ions naturally released during the process of DNA synthesis (which are then detected by a sensor). Ion Torrent devices have medium throughput and they also produce **short DNA reads** (around 600 long). Their main advantage is their size (desktop size), speed (run complete in about two hours) and their lower price per instrument and per DNA base ("letter").[3] The main competitor in this category is Illumina's desktop-sized MiSeq device.[4] (Information about other available **short-read-based NGS platforms**, such as Roche 454 Pyrosequencing, SOLID (Applied Biosystems), DNA-Nanoballs (BGI), and others can be found from various internet resources[5] and we will not analyze them here in more detail.)

Although short-read-based NGS platforms are currently standard for microbiome sequencing, another category of NGS technologies, generating lower to moderate throughput but very **long DNA reads**, is gaining popularity. Advantages of the long reads are that they typically require less computational processing (see next chapter), offer better identification of microbes at the strain-level (taxonomy), assignments to functional categories, and assembly of whole genomes.[6] Leaders in this area are the companies Pacific Biosciences (PacBio) and Oxford Nanopore. PacBio combines state-of-the-art optical technology with thousands of nanometer-sized holes on a chip, each of which fits only one single DNA molecule. This NGS technology enables super-precise continuous reading up to tens of thousands A, T, C, and G letters (currently around 30,000 bp with 10 billion reads per run). Oxford Nanopore, a spin-off company of the University of Oxford, UK, has developed instruments (some the size of the palm of a hand), which are using electrical current across a synthetic membrane filled with hundreds to thousands of nanometer-sized protein complexes forming nanometer-sized pores, similar to those in natural biological membranes. Changes in the electrical current are detected when a molecule of interest (e.g. DNA) enters the nano-pore. So far, DNA sequences longer than two million of ATCGs have been detected in one single nanopore run, meaning the complete DNA (genome) of some organisms!

Prices of NGS instruments can be as high as nearly one million dollars (NovaSeq 6000) to around one thousand dollars (Oxford Nanopore MiniION) 1. Also, prices per run, per sample, or per amount (Mb) of output can vary significantly. The final decision on which NGS platform to use depends on the desired output of an experiment (e.g. number of potential microbes, desired genome coverage, taxonomic or functional annotation, etc.) and of course, the budget of the project.

Mass Spectrometry

Besides NGS, Mass Spectrometry (MS) is another group of methods to identify known, as well as unknown bacteria in a microbiome sample. In principle, MS can be used for the analysis of any biological molecule based on the ratio between its mass and electrical charge. For bacterial identification the methods mostly used are Matrix-Assisted-Laser-Desorption/Ionisation Time-Of-Flight (MALDI-TOF) and Electro-Spray Ionization (ESI).

MALDI method is based on placing biological molecules of interest (e.g. bacterial protein) in a crystal of a known compound (matrix). A laser is then used to remove small parts of the crystal (including the molecule of interest) which are then ionized, flying in an electrostatic field, hitting a detection device. In ESI, the molecules of interest are dissolved in an organic solvent, and ionized in a small tube to which an electric current is applied, turning the molecule of interest into gas which is then detected. In both cases, the classification of bacteria is performed by comparing recorded profiles of the analyzed molecules with profiles (libraries) of known bacterial species.[7]

Except for bacterial identification, applications of MS in microbiome analysis include large-scale analysis of microbial proteins (proteomics) or their metabolites (metabolomics). In this case, molecules of interest are first separated (by liquid, gas, or electrochemical chromatography) and then detected by MS.[8]

Culturomics

We previously mentioned that more than 99 percent of all microbes on our planet cannot be cultivated (isolated and grown under specific laboratory conditions) using current methods. However, in the last few years, scientists have started to combine various methods for microbial detection, such as traditional microbiological media-based cultivation with DNA sequencing, MS, and other methods. The goal is to create a relatively cheap approach for simultaneous, automated analysis of thousands of samples (so-called "high-throughput" methods) to identify and eventually find conditions for the cultivation of so-far undetectable and/or uncultivable microbes, also known as "Microbial Dark Matter."

This group of emerging hybrid approaches is often called culturomics and will be gaining importance in the near future.[9]

As explained in Chapter 2, all the microbiomes we have isolated and analyzed might need to be stored not only on our computers but physically, for eventual repeated analysis or some practical applications such as therapy.

Further, all of the above-mentioned "high-throughput" methods generate a huge amount of data. The next logical question is how we can use these data for structural and functional analysis of human microbiomes.

This is a question we discuss directly in the following chapter.

CHAPTER 5

BIG DATA AND HOW IT'S RELEVANT

"Big data is like teenage sex: everyone talks about it, nobody really knows how to do it, everyone thinks everyone else is doing it, so everyone claims they are doing it."

—Dan Ariely, Professor, Duke University, on Facebook, 2013

THE genome of a typical bacterium such as *Escherichia coli* contains between 4.5 and 5.5 million ATCG "letters." Translated to data it will be 4.5-5.5 megabytes—not a huge amount of data—about the size of one high-resolution photo on your smartphone. However, we previously mentioned that to accurately read a genome by Next Generation Sequencing (NGS), we need to read each sequence many times. Second, when sequencing microbiomes, we often don't know how many different microbial genomes are there in our sample, so a higher sequencing "depth" (meaning more data) is recommended. Modern NGS instruments produce between a few gigabytes to up to 6 terabytes (TB) of data per single run. 6 TB equals 1.5 million high-resolution smartphone photos or around 3000 Netflix movie downloads. That's why NGS data are often classified as "big data."

I am sure many of us have assembled a jigsaw puzzle at least once. Typically, there are few hundreds or thousands of pieces and a picture according to which the puzzle should be assembled, right? For a moment imagine a billion-pieces puzzle. Difficult, right? Now, what if you need to assemble that billion-pieces puzzle but you don't have any picture? Sounds impossible? Not for the microbiome scientists. These are some of the typical tasks they face after getting their NGS data.

For these accomplishments we can thank:

a)   new generation computers,
b)   great mathematicians who invented methods for the assembly and analysis of complex series of symbols, letters, numbers,
c)   and great programmers for spending thousands of hours coding lines, trying to make scripts that will turn all of these sequences into numerical and visual outputs, out of which scientists can understand and extract meaning.

The good news is that in the last few decades, genetic, protein, and other biological sequence data have been saved at several places around the world. These databases (so-called gene, protein, and other "banks") can provide reference "pictures" for the "puzzles" mentioned above. Concretely, the computer will take each part of the microbiome sequences, compare it to all known sequences from the selected database(s) and tell you the best match. Similar to when you do your google search. However, the search can eventually return zero results, which means that we may have found a previously undiscovered microbe.

How "Big Data" Helps Analyze the Structure and Functions of Microbiomes

In the early days of DNA sequencing, to differentiate between microbes, researchers realized it was a good strategy to select genes that are conserved (not very different) among different types of microbes. The most typical example is the bacterial 16s ribosomal-RNA (16s rRNA) gene which has only a few "letters" of difference between very distant bacterial species. This kind of investigation is called "marker gene analysis." It is relatively quick and cheap compared to the sequencing of all DNA from a sample and is routinely conducted in many labs, using NGS or more traditional sequencing methods.

A more recent approach is to isolate total DNA from a sample and sequence it using one of the NGS methods described in the previous chapter. In the case of microbiomes, we will often have environmental samples (e.g. stool, skin, soil, etc.) where we don't know which microbes (i.e. which genes or genomes) we might have inside. This is why this cultivation-independent sequencing of total genetic material (DNA) in a sample is called "Metagenomics."[1] However, if our goal is specifically to sequence (and eventually assemble) complete microbial genomes in a sample, the approach is called "Whole Genome Shotgun sequencing (WGS-sequencing, or WGSS)."

Alternatively, instead of extracting DNA from the cell, we can extract RNA. As explained in Chapter 2, with some precaution, it is possible to get "good quality" RNA and store it (deep frozen) until needed. This approach in which all RNA from a sample is translated into DNA, sequenced by NGS, and analyzed is called "Transcriptomics." It tells us which microbes in the sample were actually alive, having their genes actively transcribed. Other approaches include analysis of total proteins produced by microbes in a sample ("Proteomics") or total metabolites ("Metabolomics"). For the same reason as described above for Metagenomics (environmental samples with unknown molecules), the terms "Metatranscriptomics" and "Meta-proteomics" are often used.

All of the above approaches are sometimes given the group name 'omics' technologies. The ultimate goal of applying all the "omics" in microbiome research is to learn not only about the structure of the microbial communities but also more about their functions and interactions with the host and the environment.

Higher-level Data Analysis

Besides knowing which microbes are in the sample and which functions they have, it is essential in microbiome studies to compare two or more samples, such as healthy versus diseased or drug-treated versus control. In this way, it may be possible to test if the observed condition is actually caused by the microbiota. A breakthrough in the field occurred when scientists realized that transferring gut microbiota from a diseased animal (e.g. an obese mouse) into a healthy, germ-free animal is in actuality transferring the disease. Since then, a similar approach has been used for various other diseases.[2]

Comparing different microbiome samples can be quite complicated and includes various questions. Let us take a few examples. How abundant is one microbial species in each sample and how does that differ between different samples? How many different species (also known as diversity) are there in each sample and how does that differ between samples A, B, …? How related are observed species in one sample and between samples (phylogeny)? How different (or diverse) are functions which species in each sample can perform (functional diversity)?[3]

In addition, microbiome studies often collect various descriptions of the data such as date, time, type of the sample (human, animal, plant, environmental), geographical location, age, sex, ethnicity, diet, disease state, medication intake, season, weather conditions, etc. These are called "metadata" and can be very relevant for subsequent analyses.[4]

To find eventual patterns between samples and answer the above questions, researchers are using various, often advanced, statistical methods. To extract the meaning from the big, multi-dimensional data, visualization methods are also needed. Examples include heat maps, graphical networks, and others. Machine-learning (ML) approaches are becoming very popular to cross-analyze microbiome samples, including metadata. For example, ML methods can be used to develop new microbiome therapies, predict therapy outcomes, or diagnose health conditions based on microbiomes.[5] A number of microbiome companies are already routinely employing ML in their workflows and others (such as Ardigen, Biome Diagnostics, Eagle Genomics, or REM Analytics) have become specialized providers of the "data-mining" services to other microbiome researchers.

PART III

IN HEALTH AND DISEASE

CHAPTER 6

WHAT IS A 'HEALTHY MICROBIOME'?

Is having a diverse gut microbial community the key to a healthy microbiome? Are there specific gut microbial species that represent hallmarks of being healthy? These are just a few of the questions that scientists are trying to understand in deciphering the microbiome traits that support health and the normal ranges of these traits in healthy populations. Understanding the traits of a healthy microbiome would enable healthy people to remain healthy and improve the health of diseased individuals.

Let's Define Healthy Microbiome

From a microbial ecology perspective, a healthy microbiome should have these two traits, resistance and resilience. Resistance is defined as the ability to resist perturbations and resilience is defined as the ability to return to a healthy or equilibrium state after the perturbations.[1] For example, after an antibiotic treatment, a healthy gut microbiome generally recovers to its previous state after a few weeks or months.[2] This indicates that the gut microbiome is not in a single static state but rather in a dynamic equilibrium. The gut microbiome within an individual is constantly changing due to external and internal factors, gaining, and losing species over time, some microbial taxa having different stabilities, and some remaining in the gut for many years.[3]

Early microbiome research was focused on discovering which microorganisms define a healthy microbiome, a set of microbial families which are present in all healthy people.[4] But large microbiome-focused studies, investigating the composition and function of the microbiome in a healthy population,[5] have shown that microbiomes, especially in the gut, show a large degree of variation between individuals, and thus no single gut microbiome configuration can be defined as healthy. Therefore, the theory of a core microbiome, a set of microbial taxa that would universally be present in healthy individuals, has been rendered unlikely. Despite large compositional diversity between individuals, also known as inter-individual variability, and the resilience of the gut microbiome in an individual, also referred to as intra-individual variability, the function of the gut microbiome is less diverse and highly conserved. The function refers to what the microorganisms are doing in the gastrointestinal tract, for example, what substances they metabolize and what they produce. This suggests that functionality and not the composition of the microbiome is better in distinguishing a normal from an abnormal microbiome.

Furthermore, gut microbiome diversity has been linked to human health,[6] but diversity alone cannot be used to define a healthy microbiome. As mentioned above, the presence or absence of specific microbial families should be carefully used in distinguishing between a healthy and diseased microbiome. For example, two beneficial genera, *Bifidobacterium* and *Faecalibacterium*, are negatively correlated with one another. This relationship indicates that one of these genera is dominant and can outcompete the other one for the same nutrients. The same relationship has been observed between the families *Lachnospiraceae* and *Ruminococcaceae*; both are considered beneficial microbial families that can ferment dietary fibers and produce butyrate, one of the most important short-chain fatty acids (SCFAs).[7] Moreover, it became clear that studying the microbiome at the strain level matters. Microbiome studies are often focused on studying the different microbial species without distinguishing between the different strains. For example, *Bifidobacterium longum* is a microbial species present in the gastrointestinal tract, but if we are to look at the strains level there are more than 400 different strains of *Bifidobacterium longum*,[8] and as you will see in the probiotic chapters, not all microbial strains are the same. Another example is *Escherichia coli* (*E. coli*), one of the most well-known and studied microbes, which is also a commensal living in the gut. There are different strains of *E. coli*, some can promote food digestion and have probiotic actions, while other strains are pathogens and can cause infections.[9] The same is true for many other microbial strains being associated with beneficial functions but also correlated with diseases, some examples are *Prevotella copri*,[10] *Faecalibacterium prausnitzii*,[11] and *Eubacterium rectale*.[12]

Strongly Influenced by Internal and External Factors

Lifestyle, diet, and medication are only a few of the factors that have a huge impact on the gut microbiome. Taking into consideration the age of an individual, we can discern different factors that will influence the microbiome over an individual's lifetime.

At birth, infants acquire from their mother important microbes as they pass through the birth canal. That is why, infants that are born via C-section might miss out on valuable microbes that are passed from the mother to the infant during birth and they might be at higher risk of developing diseases later on in life, such as allergies, asthma, obesity, and diabetes.[13] This is because an infant's first years of life are important not only for the infant's growth and development of the organs but also for the development of a healthy microbiome. Any perturbations happening in the first year of life, such as exposure to antibiotics, can have a detrimental effect on the development of the microbiome. In the first years of life, the developing microbiome plays an important role in educating the immune system, especially in teaching it how to distinguish between good microbes and bad microbes, such as pathogens.[14]

Another important factor that has been shown to have a strong effect on the development of the microbiome in infants, is the mode of feeding. Breast milk not only contains important nutrients for the infant and immune factors to protect the infant against pathogens, it also contains important microbes that are being transferred to the infant.[15] Furthermore, human milk contains human milk oligosaccharides (HMOs), which are chains of sugars that are not digested by human enzymes but are food for the microbes, especially for the *Bifidobacterium* and *Lactobacillus* genera. HMOs thus modulate the microbiome and help the development of a healthy microbiome. Moreover, HMOs play a protective role in diarrhea and infections in infants.[16]

One more important factor that has been proven to have a strong impact on the development of the microbiome in infants is the environment. Children that are raised together with animals, especially dogs, and those that are raised close to farm animals, are at lower risk of developing allergies and asthma compared to children that are raised in urban environments.[17] The reason is that having a dog or other animals in the proximity of a growing child will increase the diversity of the microbes to which the child is being exposed, thus having a beneficial effect on the growth and health of that child. These are only some of the factors that influence the development of a healthy microbiome early in life. After three years, a child's gut microbiome starts resembling that of an adult.[18]

In adults, the changes observed in the microbiome are mainly driven by lifestyle and environment. A large population study conducted in Israel has shown that the environment contributes to 20–25 percent of the observed variance in the microbiome composition between individuals.[19] Some of the factors identified were diet, medication, and anthropometric measurements, such as age, sex, and BMI. The effect of drugs and the interaction between the drugs and microbiome have been described in detail in Chapter 15 under Pharmaco-microbiomics. Lifestyle is another factor that strongly influences the microbiome; for example, sedentary lifestyle, smoking, consumption of alcohol, exposure to stress, and unhealthy eating habits are only a few of the factors that have been so far studied for their negative effect on the human body and the US microbiome.[20]

Diet is a well-known factor that strongly shapes the gut microbiome. After all, it is true what they say; we are what we eat, and so is the microbiome that is shaped by the food we ingest. In the long history of the human race, people's eating habits have gradually changed. Looking back at the first humans, their diet was mainly plants and berries. During the farming period, the diet underwent another change when people started eating grains and consuming animal products, such as milk and dairy, and meat. The industrialized era brought not only new complex processes to manufacture our food, but also additional additives and flavors that are added to foods to extend the shelf-life of products and increase the taste. Studies of indigenous populations who have a traditional rural or hunter-gatherer lifestyle, resembling those of our ancestors, have shown that industrialization led to a loss of gut microbial diversity.[21] One of the potential culprits of microbial diversity loss is the lack of fibers in Western diets. The Hadza hunter-gatherers living in Tanzania consume between 100–150 grams of dietary fibers every day, while a typical person in Europe or US eats less than 20 grams of fibers per day. Furthermore, their gut microbiome contains high levels of *Prevotella* species, well-known microbes able to digest different types of fiber, while these bacterial taxa seem to be missing in individuals from industrialized countries.[22] Given the fact that gut microbial diversity has been linked with health and that food in the industrialized era is leading to a gradual loss of microbial diversity and species, there is a strong link between western diet (such as processed foods with excess fat, high sugar content, additives, and little amounts of dietary fibers and micronutrients) and high incidence rate of diseases which are increasing in developed countries.[23] Therefore, understanding how dietary choices influence the microbiome and how they can lead to disease is important for preventive measures to reduce the risk of diseases and modulate a healthy gut microbiome via dietary interventions.

The Balanced Gut Microbiome—Eubiosis and Dysbiosis

A healthy host-microbiome interaction, also known as homeostasis, has to be maintained for the optimal performance of metabolic and immune functions and prevention of disease development. The human body is in continuous contact with trillions of microorganisms and maintains a state of homeostasis by tightly controlling the microbiome through immune responses and other processes. The development of a healthy microbiome is crucial, as the first interactions between the microorganisms and the developing immune system will determine the proper function of the immune system distinguishing between friends, beneficial microbes, or foes, harmful microbes.[24]

In the gut, homeostasis is maintained through controlling the anaerobiosis, a state without oxygen, and the immune response toward gut microbiota. The host minimizes the amount of oxygen resulting from the mucosal surface by maintaining the colon cells in a state of hypoxia (less than 1 percent of oxygen being present). The reason behind it is that in the absence of oxygen the anaerobic microorganisms in the gut will ferment carbohydrates to short-chain fatty acids (SCFAs), which are an important source of nutrients for the cells in the gut. In the presence of oxygen, these organisms will switch to using oxygen instead of fermentation resulting in digestion of the SCFAs to carbon dioxide, which has been shown to interfere with host nutrition.[25] Therefore, maintaining the balance between beneficial microbes and harmful microbes is important for the proper function of both the microbiome and the host.

Eubiosis is defined as the balanced host-microbiome interaction, while dysbiosis is often defined as a disbalance in the gut microbiota and is associated with diseases.[26] The eubiotic and dysbiotic states of the gut microbiome are strongly associated with gut homeostasis.

External factors such as poor diet, lack of exercise, stress, and taking antibiotics or other drugs can cause a disbalance in your body and in your microbiome, which will affect the gut homeostasis leading to certain digestive problems, such as diarrhea and constipation, but can also lead to more threatening infections or diseases.[27] Therefore, understanding the factors that can lead to dysbiosis and how they affect gut homeostasis is important in restoring eubiosis during perturbations and in disease, and how the power of the microbiome can be harvested to maintain a healthy host-microbiome interaction.

Search for the Missing Pieces—Future Perspectives

As already discussed in this chapter, numerous factors have to be considered in defining a healthy microbiome and how we can translate this information in a clinical context to prevent diseases and maintain a healthy status. Although we have gained a better understanding of what gut microbiomes look like and what might be their functions, we are far from identifying the key components of a microbiome that are essential for our wellbeing. Defining a healthy microbiome based on the microbial composition or function alone might not be enough and the focus will have to be directed towards the interactions between the microbiome and the host, especially on uncovering the factors that are influencing this interaction, and the role the microbiome plays in health and disease.

We are yet to uncover all the internal and external factors that influence our microbiome, a more diverse population has to be considered to understand the loss of microbial diversity encountered in the industrialized world and how to prevent it or even restore the microbiome to a healthier state. Most of the studies to date are focused on people from well-developed countries, such as the United States, European countries, and China and only a handful of studies have looked at indigenous populations. Thankfully, initiatives such as the Global Microbiome Conservancy (GMbC) will help us in closing this information gap. The GMbC is aiming to create a biobank of human microbiomes from a wide variety of human populations worldwide, especially indigenous people and other under-represented communities.[28] A large, more global dataset of different microbiome configurations would help in better understanding what a normal microbiome looks like in healthy individuals, and would make it easier to recognize diseased-like perturbations.

Lastly, with an ever-growing development of new methodologies to study the microbiome and its interactions with the host, future microbiome studies should include various microbiome-analysis techniques. Using various techniques would give us a more comprehensive picture of what happens in our bodies and how are the microbes communicating with each other and with the human host.

CHAPTER 7

CO-DEPENDENT WORLD OF OUR IMMUNE SYSTEM AND MICROBIOMES

OUR immune system is a complex network of organs, white blood cells, proteins, and chemicals. It is divided into two interconnected parts: the *natural* (aka "innate") immune system that we are born with, and the *adaptive* immune system, that we develop when our body is exposed to microbes or chemicals released by microbes or other foreign molecules.

The innate immune system is the first to react as it helps to create physical barriers that protect the body. When an invader, a microorganism, is detected, this type of immune system cells surrounds and covers it. The invader is finally eliminated within the immune system cells, called phagocytes. The innate immune system provides i) protection by the skin and mucous membranes, and ii) by immune system cells (defense cells) and proteins.

However, if the innate immune system is unable to eradicate the germs, the adaptive immune system takes over. It is developed to directly target the microorganisms generating the infection. To accomplish this, it must first recognize the microbes. This implies that it is slower to react than the innate immune system, but it is more effective when it does. It also has the benefit of being able to "remember" pathogens, so that the adaptive immune system may react faster the next time known pathogens are addressed. This memory is also the explanation for why some illnesses can only be contracted once in a lifetime, with the body becoming "immune" thereafter. The adaptive immune system may take a few days to respond the first time when it comes in touch with the pathogen, but responds promptly the next time. The second infection is frequently not recognized, or is much weaker. The adaptive immune system consists of specialized cells, also known as *lymphocytes*. There are two types of lymphocytes: *B-cells* and *T-cells*. B-cells produce proteins known as *antibodies* (or immunoglobulins) in response to a specific *antigen*. An antigen is typically a foreign substance that causes the body to make an immune response. Antibodies combine chemically with antigens according to the lock and key principle, helping the body to recognize and neutralize aliens such as bacteria or viruses. Certain B-cells also have the ability to "remember" contact with an antigen. T cells play different roles in the adaptive immune system, either by directly killing other infected cells ("T-killer" cells), by supporting other cells involved in immune response ("T-helper" cells), or by regulating the immune response so that other immune cells do not react to own body's cells ("T-regs").

However, most of the microbial cells in human microbiota are NOT recognized by our immune system as aliens. An increasing number of scientific reports point to the existence of continuous and reciprocal communication between the immune system and microbiota, defined as "microbiota-inflammation" or "microbiota-immunity axis."[1] Indeed, as we will see, microbiota and the immune system are deeply linked.

Like Two Sides of the Same Coin

Certain bacterial members of our microbiota use the food we supply them, without providing us any benefit or doing harm. These are called *commensal* bacteria. Other bacteria also use food from us, but provide us some beneficial chemicals in return. They are called *symbiotic* bacteria. Our immune system has evolved different methods to tolerate both kinds of bacteria, maintaining a state of balance with them. In fact, human microbiota does not induce an immune response capable of causing inflammation (pro-inflammatory) in a normal healthy condition. However, when this delicate equilibrium is impaired, due to changes in environmental factors (such as unbalanced diet, antibiotic use, or changes in geography), it can lead to the overgrowth of other types of harmful or disease-causing microorganisms (aka "pathogens") and thus in an altered immune response.

This mutual interplay has been currently linked to a number of "non-communicable" gastrointestinal pathologies, such as celiac disease, inflammatory bowel disease (IBD), or extra-intestinal conditions including rheumatic diseases, neurodegenerative disorders, metabolic syndromes, and tumors. In addition, the microbiota-immunity axis has been currently studied to better understand the pathogenesis, prognosis, and severity of both COVID-19 disease and Long COVID-19 syndrome.[2]

Furthermore, the microbiota–immunity axis is affected by a combination of environmental factors, which have a greater influence than the host genetics. Diet, antibiotic usage, and environmental pollution are all possible drivers of inflammatory and autoimmune illnesses (a condition in which the body's immune system mistakes its own healthy tissues as foreign and attacks them). Understanding regulation of the human microbiota and its influence on the immune system as a trigger of disease, however, is still in its infancy but let's try to explain a few facts that are known.

Microbiota Helps Development of Our Immune System

The first colonization of the inner lining of the human gut (mucosa) by microbes happens in early life and it is crucial for the "education" of the immune system.[3] Microbial colonization occurs after delivery, mainly originating from the contact between the newborn oral cavity and the maternal vaginal microbiota and is influenced by a number of factors, including delivery mode: the gut microbiota of naturally born babies is different from those born by cesarean section. However, according to some recent research, gut colonization by microbiota may begin even earlier. While the conventional hypothesis was that a newborn's intestines are sterile until delivery, new research showed a microbial population already present in the meconium (the first feces of the newborn) of certain prematurely born kids.[4]

The most critical events in the development of the infant's immunity occur during the early life years, when further microbial colonization continues, before stabilizing as an "adult" microbiota around the age of 3 years. Most of the information on the modulation of the immune system by the microbiota has been derived from experiments on previously mentioned germ-free (GF) animals, born without microorganisms living in or on them. Indeed, the lack of bacteria in GF mice is linked to significant changes in the immunological function of the intestine. Regarding GF mice, when they undergo microbial colonization, it is possible to observe several effects on the immune system.

Of note, lymphocytes that are located in the gastrointestinal system recognize antigens (for example on the surface of a microbial cell), rapidly responding by the release of mediators of inflammation known as cytokines, destroying the target cells. In detail, cytokines are various chemicals (such as interferon, interleukin, and growth factors) that are secreted by special cells of the immune system and have an effect on other cells. They are crucial in controlling the growth and activity of other immune system cells. In addition, extracellular metabolites generated by commensal gut microorganisms can regulate B-cells in the gut, influencing the production of antibodies.

In this context, the interaction between microbiota and the immune system in early life can have a high impact on the maturation and function of the immune system of an organism, contributing to immune balance and susceptibility to inflammatory and infectious conditions later in life. Nevertheless, the pathways behind these interplays are currently largely unexplored. More investigations on the long-term effects of a disruption of microbiota (dysbiosis) during pregnancy, the early years of life on adult immunity, and the risk of immune-mediated diseases are required.

What Happens in Healthy Status?

The "gut mucosa" is the upper layer of the intestine, usually exposed to bacteria. It represents a good model to study host–microbiota interactions through the microbiota–immunity axis. In fact, when a huge and dynamic commensal bacterial population occupies the gut, the intestinal-associated immune system is able to tolerate it while, at the same time, it also sustains immune responses against pathogenic infection or commensal infiltration into the other internal body parts without bacteria.

In a healthy state, the host's immune response to the intestinal microbiota is strictly localized to the mucosal surface, the slimy layer where a thick mucus separates the surface layer of gut cells (epithelium) from the microbiota.[5] Concomitantly, the mucus barrier physically limits the ability of microbial cells to provoke an immune response by contacting immune cells in the gut wall.[6] Moreover, the tight junctions between mucosa cells regulate the translocation of material from the internal intestine (such as food molecules, minerals, and water) to the bloodstream or other organs.

Simply, if our gut mucosa layer is healthy and strong, it prevents the leak of unwanted molecules or antigens, thus preventing immune response and inflammation. Happy system, healthy life!

Gut mucosa is barrier that prevents direct contact of microbes inside the gut with the blood and immune system. In a healthy state, gut mucosa consists of a thick layer of mucus (slime) and tightly connected cells of the gut wall. If the gut barrier becomes leaky (e.g. by damaging mucus layer or by loosening of the cell-to-cell junctions) microbes can get recognized by the immune cell in the gut wall causing local inflammation. Eventually, microbial molecules can enter into the bloodstream causing systemic effects and potentially a disease.

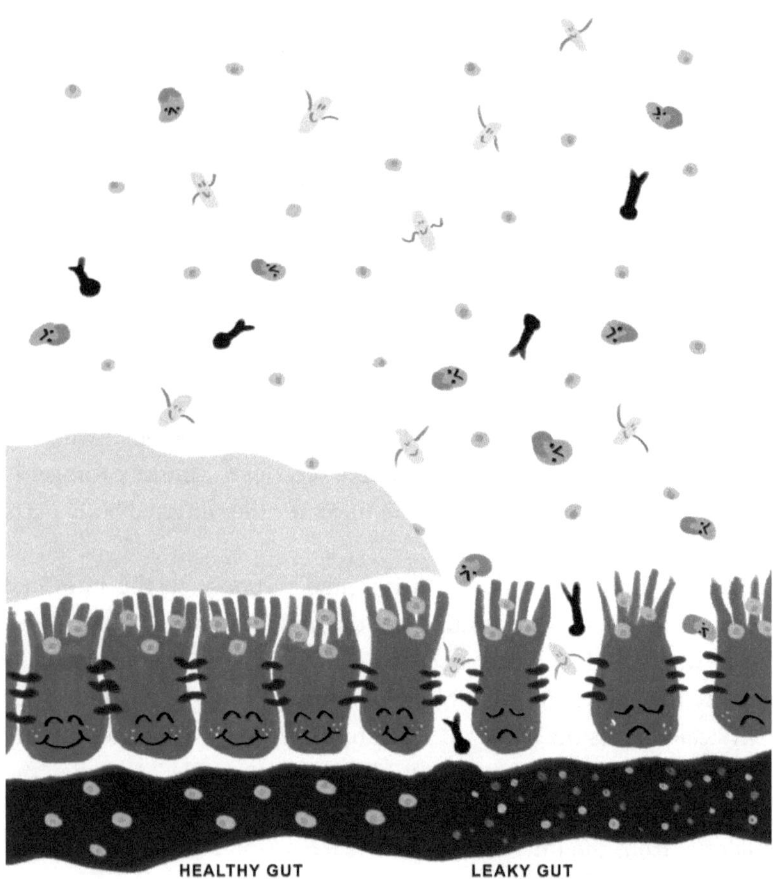

Fig. 7.1 Gut mucosa is barrier that prevents direct contact of microbes inside the gut with the blood and immune system

Microbiota Crosstalk Prevents Pathogens

As mentioned above, the innate immune system is the body's initial line of defense against pathogens. It responds to all pathogens and foreign chemicals in the same way, which is why it is frequently referred to as the "non-specific" immune system. For example, the innate immune system ensures that germs that enter the skin through a minor wound are recognized and eliminated on the spot within a few hours. However, this mechanism has only a limited ability to prevent pathogens from spreading. In the mutual interplay between microbiota and innate immune response, several immune "actors" are involved. First, the antimicrobial peptides secreted by specialized cells in the gut mucosa (called Paneth cells)[7] can interact with the gut microbiota, affecting its composition.[8] Second, proteins of the immune cells called pattern recognition receptors (PRRs) identify microbial signals (patterns), triggering an immune response. Third, a protein called NOD1 (nucleotide-binding oligomerization domain-containing protein) in the cells of the gut mucosa can sense small molecules produced by the gut bacteria, stimulating the development of lymphoid tissues (places where immune cells organize and develop). Furthermore, large protein complexes called "inflammasomes" assemble in response to infection- or stress-related stimuli and activate an immune response. Inflammasome activation may be caused by a wide range of pathogenic microbes and, in general, support host defense by activating fast inflammatory processes and limiting pathogen reproduction.

On the other hand, B-cells are important mediators of gut balance because they produce a wide range of antibodies (immunoglobulins) that are sensitive to commensal microflora.[9] IgA, for example, are immune globulins secreted by the human gut, serving an essential function in the structuring of gut bacterial populations.[10] Another example of microbiota regulation of adaptive immune responses is previously mentioned T-killer lymphocytes, whose activity is crucial in the elimination of intracellular pathogens and tumor cells. Also, numerous researches published over the last decade have provided a comprehensive picture of the interplay between gut microbiota and the regulatory T cells (T-regs) that block the actions of some other types of lymphocytes, to keep the immune system from becoming over-active.

Can Dysregulation of Microbiota-Immunity Interaction Cause Diseases?

In genetically susceptible individuals, atypical relationships between the microbiota and the host immune response can result in the development of complicated immunological-mediated diseases and health disorders. Here, we will list a few.

Rheumatoid Arthritis

Rheumatoid arthritis (RA) is a systemic chronic autoimmune inflammatory disease characterized by the destruction of bone in multiple joints and auto-antibody production such as rheumatoid factor and in particular, anti-citrullinated protein antibodies, the most powerful and early diagnostic markers.[11] During inflammation, the shape of certain proteins is significantly changed, so that they are seen as foreign (antigens) by the immune system, triggering an auto-immune response. The RA pathogenesis is currently unclear, however, genetic, microbiota, and environmental factors have been implicated. Regarding microbiota, new-onset RA patients[12] display decrease and increase in richness of particular gut bacteria.[13] Moreover, the periodontal infection (infection of the gum and bones around teeth) by the bacterium *Porphyromonas gingivalis* is also involved in exacerbating inflammatory arthritis.[14] Of note, periodontitis is characterized by a chronic inflammation caused by oral bacteria and blood cells infiltration with progressive damage to the tooth. The idea that oral microbiota is involved in RA development is supported by the high frequency of periodontal inflammatory disorders in RA patients.[15] Another proof of the link between RA and oral inflammation is the evidence that the treatment of a periodontal disease may improve RA symptoms.[16] However, future research is needed to identify the impact of RA therapy on the microbiota and the causative role of microbiota changes in regulating rheumatoid arthritis.

Cardiometabolic Diseases

As we will see in the next chapter, chronic low-grade inflammation is thought to be a defining feature of metabolic illnesses such as diabetes and obesity, as well as associated diseases such as atherosclerosis and non-alcoholic fatty liver disease (NAFLD). Crosstalk between immune cells and parenchymal organ tissue (the main tissue of an organ consisting of actively dividing cells) is crucial in the physiology of metabolic disorders in highly active organs such as the liver or adipose tissue.[17] Growing data suggest that microbiota metabolites can enter the systemic circulation and promote "metabolic inflammation," a term used to describe the combined simultaneous disorder of immune and metabolic pathways.[18] Several linkages between the host immune system and gut bacteria have been implicated in type-1 diabetes. Furthermore, the interplay between the microbiota and immune system is important in obesity. Atherosclerosis and its consequences are among the most dangerous phases of cardiometabolic illness. In detail, the trimethylamine N-oxide (TMAO), a molecule generated from certain food types by the gut microbiota (which we will discuss in the chapter about microbiome and nutrition), has been related to atherosclerotic heart disease in both mice and humans.[19]

Other cardiometabolic diseases (heart disease linked to metabolic disorders) such as atrial fibrillation (AF), are frequently associated with heart failure (HF), a clinical syndrome caused by structural and/or functional heart abnormalities and characterized by fatigue due to insufficient pumping of the blood to the organ systems. It has been defined as a global pandemic since it affects more than 26 million people worldwide and to date, it is one of the few cardiovascular conditions whose prevalence continues to rise.[20] Of note, AF and HF synergistically contribute to determining the state of weakness and increased mortality (especially at an advanced age). Due to the loss of appetite, they can also lead to undernutrition, which may worsen and progress toward an inflammation-related wasting process affecting all body compartments including bone, fat, and skeletal muscle. Undernourished AF and HF patients enter a vicious cycle "of undernutrition, inflammation, weakness,"[21] which leads to further deterioration of nutritional status. Chronic or acute disease-related malnutrition is linked with chronic or acute inflammation that in turn is associated with reduced complexity of the gut microbiota and its metabolites. The microbiota plays an important role in the absorption, storage, and expenditure of energy obtained from dietary intake. Since inflammation is closely related to the health of intestinal microbiota, shaping the gut microbiota composition with a probiotic-based food, specifically enriched with key nutrients, could be an efficacious and safe approach to break this cycle and improve cognitive functioning and skeletal muscle mass. In this context, the AMBROSIA project[22] is the first study that simultaneously considers nutritional profile and a related intervention, inflammatory biomarkers and intestinal microbiota. AMBROSIA aims to develop an innovative food product to prevent undernutrition in HF and AF older patients, as a new chocolate AMBROSIA bar containing a specific mix of probiotic strains specifically addressed to the microbiome–immunity axis.

Inflammatory Bowel Disease

Inflammatory bowel disease (IBD), which comprises Crohn's disease (CD) and ulcerative colitis (UC), is characterized by chronic inflammation of the gastrointestinal tract, leading to bowel damage. Between them, CD is a multifactorial intestinal disorder, which causes major life-long disability. The time of CD onset is usually during young adulthood and it is characterized by periods of remission, a temporary diminution of the severity of disease and relapse, and the return of an illness after a period of improvement. CD pathogenesis is still unclear and the reasons for repeated (recurrent) disease after a surgical intervention remain speculative. Recent studies have indicated that a complex interplay of genetic, microbial, and environmental factors generates abnormal intestinal innate immunity. This imbalanced innate immunity may be a central early mechanism, followed by dysregulated adaptive immune responses, contributing to the typical damages (lesions) of the gut mucosa.[23] Furthermore, the collapse of the gut mucosa (intestinal barrier) allows bacteria to move into the mucosal layer, generating host immune (inflammatory) responses and tissue destruction.[24] Moreover, numerous studies have shown that the complex regulatory mechanisms associated with mucosal immunity against microbiota can lead to an excessive inflammatory response, contributing to CD.[25] Multiple other lines of evidence point toward the central roles of gut microbiota in CD development. Few studies have evaluated microbiota during surgeries to identify bacteria involved in CD and showed that the intestinal microbiota underwent major changes following surgery (with differences between patients with or without repeated disease). A recent study also analyzed the immune system of different gut layers and microbiota composition in the small gut.[26] They observed a different distribution of inflammatory molecules and microbiota composition within diseased and adjacent healthy gut tissue layers, and also between patients after the first operation and patients with multiple operations. These results give insight into the dynamics of the gut microbiota–immune axis in CD patients, potentially leading to the detection of new diagnostic markers.

Cancer

Different studies in GF animals associated with bacteria have revealed evidence for tumor-promoting effects of the microbiota in spontaneous and genetically-linked cancers in several organs, including skin, colon, liver, breast, and lungs.[27] There are also data showing the contrary view that gut microbiota has a central role in limiting chemically induced injury and proliferative responses that lead to cancer development in germ-free animals.[28] Anyway, inflammatory responses induced by bacteria were demonstrated to enhance cancer progression.[29] For example, if the gut mucosa becomes "leaky", some bacteria and/or their toxins can pass into the bloodstream and to the rest of the body, causing inflammation which contributes to the development, progression, and treatment of cancer. It remains unclear whether commensal bacteria affect inflammation in the immediate tumor environment. An increasing number of studies demonstrated the role of inflammation in establishing conditions that can deeply alter local immune responses and thus, tissue balance. In particular, it is well documented that inflammatory mediators are involved in a progressive interplay between the immune cells and tissue cells undergoing cancer transformation.[30]

Normally the components of the adaptive immune system are silent; however, when activated, these components 'adapt' to the presence of infectious agents or abnormal cells by creating potent mechanisms to neutralize or eliminate them. On the other hand, the adaptive immune system is essential for the establishment of complex bacterial communities in the gut. One of the main mechanisms by which a dysfunctional microbiota can indirectly promote tumor growth is T-helper lymphocytes called "Th17" cells. Namely, commensal microbiota actively shapes the intestinal T-cell responses that promote balance in healthy conditions. However, in response to bacterial or fungal infections, Th17 cells can become pathogenic and induce chronic inflammation and autoimmune diseases. The microbiota has been recently shown to modulate anti-cancer immunotherapy responses. Of note, cancer immunotherapy is the stimulation of the immune system to treat cancer, improving upon the immune system's natural ability to fight the disease.[31] We will discuss more about this in the part about microbiome-based therapies.

Microbiota-Inflammation in Covid-19 Disease

All the current evidence pointing to the links between COVID-19 disease and the host microbiota involves the activation of inflammatory processes and regulation of the innate and adaptive immune response. Indeed, a strong immune response characterized by the secretion of large amounts of cytokines can create a hyper-inflammation status called "cytokine-storm," which is a life-threatening condition. Also, as we will see soon, the gut microbiota affects lung health through the so-called "gut-lung axis," involving immuno-regulatory mechanisms. This mutual interaction is created mainly by immune cells and intestinal bacteria, suggesting the existence of tight crosstalk between enteric and lung microbiota. In other words, the gut microbiota can influence the immune response in the lung environment and vice versa, also involving intestinal microbial metabolites which can potentially damage the lung tissue. Lung damage further increases the production of pro-inflammatory cytokines and promotes the presence of the microbial species known to worsen the severity of the SARS-CoV-2 infection.

The impact of the gut microbiota-immunity axis on SARS CoV-2 has been documented in several studies. For example, in the study of Yeoh et al[32] among hospitalized COVID-19 patients, the inflammatory markers were significantly related to changes in the gut microbiota profile. In addition, in patients with a severe form of COVID-19 disease, a recent study found a considerable increase in permeability of the gut mucosa, implying a so-called "leaky gut" condition. It's also worth noting that the crosstalk between the gut and the lung can indicate the influence of SARS-CoV-2 infection on the gut microflora structure. In fact, COVID-19 patients have a different composition of fecal bacteria than healthy controls and the gut microbiota composition pattern was positively correlated with an increased amount of pro-inflammatory cytokines.[33] Individual susceptibility to COVID-19 is likely to be influenced by the pre-existing health (and microbiota) condition and changes after SARS-CoV-2 infection. In fact, the virus replication triggers the release of mediators of inflammation, leading to the development of a severe acute immune response with increased gut permeability. On the other hand, the "leaky gut" allows the translocation of microbial toxins and metabolites to the systemic circulation further fueling inflammation. Vicious cycle, isn't it?

Graft vs Host Disease

Graft-versus-host disease (GvHD) is a common side effect of transplantation of blood-forming cells (usually from the bone marrow), also known as Hematopoietic Cell Transplantation or HCT. It happens when the immune cells from the donor attack cells of the recipient, causing inflammation in the whole body. GvHD has a negative effect on the recipient's quality of life and can be potentially lethal. On the other hand, HCT is a life-saving treatment for managing hematological malignancies such as leukemia and lymphoma, as well as preserving bone marrow activity in patients with conditions linked with abnormal formation of blood cells.

The field around the microbiome and GvHD is rapidly developing. Indeed, GvHD most typically involves microbiota-rich tissues such as the intestinal tract, mouth, and skin, as well as the liver (which is seeded with bacterial molecules from the portal circulation). Many reports on animal and human experiments show that the gut microbiota composition is linked to the risk of GvHD, but the mechanisms involved remain unknown. Interestingly in well-controlled experimental systems, the animal studies provide compelling evidence that microbes play a role in modulating GvHD. For example, using advanced molecular methods[1], it has been demonstrated that depletion of *Lactobacillus* species was associated with worsening of GvHD, whereas replacement of lactobacilli was associated with protection. Regarding human studies, various reports have reported decreased bacterial diversity in GvHD patients.[2, 3]

So, manipulating the gut microbiota is one promising avenue for preventing or treating this common condition, and targeted application of antibiotics during transplantation may help preserve the microbiota while modulating immune responses to benefit the host. Some companies, such as Maat Pharma are already developing microbiome-based therapies for GvHD.

To conclude, more research on microbial interaction is needed to investigate the functions of microbiota in immune system regulation, as well as in health and pathologic conditions. Moreover, the microbiome variability existing among individuals and its associated ecological complexity poses a significant experimental challenge, but it also presents an opportunity for microbiota research by allowing the use of artificial intelligence, such as machine learning, in deciphering individualized microbiome profiles that impact human health. As a result, predicting "personalized" host immune responses based on these gut microbiota profiles would be exciting, potentially facilitating the development of tailored microbiota-targeted therapeutics for immunological illnesses.

MICROBIAL GUT-BRAIN AXIS, METABOLIC AND GUT CONDITIONS CONNECTED TO THE GUT MICROBIOME

Communication Between Gut Microbiome and the Brain

THE connection between the brain and our digestive tract is so intuitive that it doesn't need any explanation. How many times have we heard that someone is emotionally "sick" or has a "gut feeling." Our favorite is "so shit scared that have to quickly go to the toilet." The gut and nervous system connection are as old as the first gut itself, which is some 550 million years.[1] To give us a time scale, our brains are 500 times younger than the first gut, and only in the last twenty years have we begun to understand the links between our gut microbes and our brain.

Experiments with the germ-free (GF) mice have shown serious defects in the normal development of their brains, nerve cells, and behavior as adults. Interestingly, some of these symptoms could have been reverted by the introduction of certain microbial species in the gut. Observed mental effects in humans after infection or antibiotic treatment, also indicated gut–brain connection and gave birth to a whole new field of research.[2]

How Do Gut Microbes Communicate to Our Brain?

There are three main routes of communication of our gut microbes to our brain: via the immune system, bloodstream, and nervous system. To understand this, we need to understand a little bit of our body's anatomy. The walls of our guts are built of cells acting like bricks in a wall, joined by organic "cement." Normally, this prevents the passing through of unwanted foreign molecules into our blood. If the "cement" gets loose and the wall leaky, molecules (such as bacterial lipopolysaccharides [LPS]) can pass through, giving an alarm signal to our *immune system* to start a defense response by triggering inflammation. On the other hand, the immune system and the brain are also interlinked on several levels, details of which would make this book even thicker.

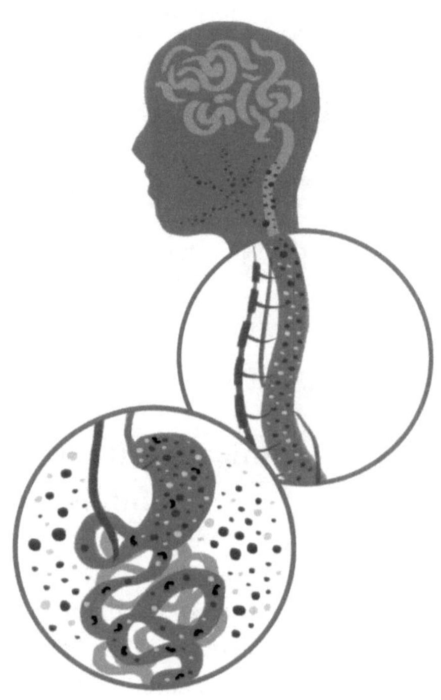

Fig. 8.1 Communication between gut and brain is bidirectional. Chemicals produced by the gut microbes act on brain via blood , nervous system and immune system. Inversely, chemicals produced by brain affect gut and gut microbes, directly or indirectly

Importantly, some of the "bricks" in the gut wall are different from others. These are special cells, called enteroendocrine cells (EEC) and enterochromaffin (EC) cells. They detect chemicals secreted by our gut microbes and, as a result of this "talk," secrete other chemicals (such as peptides, hormones, or neurotransmitters) which communicate to the nerve endings or are secreted into the *bloodstream*, traveling directly to the brain. Nerve cells of our gut walls have their own nerve system (also known as the enteric nerve system) which tells our guts how and when to move. Like big cables, other larger *nerve bundles* connect our guts to the brain. One set of cables goes through the spinal cord. Another, important big nerve, is called the "vagus" (meaning "wanderer" in Latin) which communicates both directly to our gut cells and via the enteric nerve system.

Irritable Bowel Syndrome: It isn't Just Your Tummy

Irritable bowel syndrome (IBS) happens in people who experience strong psychological trauma. It includes abdominal pain, diarrhea, constipation, or a combination thereof, and also disruption of the gut microbiota (dysbiosis). Low levels of certain chemicals produced by gut microbes, such as short-chain fatty acids (SCFAs) are typical for IBS patients, suggesting a microbial link. IBS is often seen in combination with depression and other severe neuro-psychiatric conditions. Cortisol is a hormone produced by adrenal glands when the brain signals them stress conditions. Cortisol makes gut walls leaky, causing inflammation, thus making symptoms of anxiety and depression even worse. On the other hand, serotonin is a hormone that regulates anxiety, and the majority of it in the body is produced by the above-mentioned enterochromaffin cells.[3] Gut dysbiosis occurs both in depression and general anxiety disorders. When microbiomes from depressed human patients are inserted in rats, they also start to show symptoms of depression. In humans, it has been shown that special strains of live bacteria or their metabolites can reduce stress and alleviate the symptoms of depression. These kinds of pro- and prebiotics (see Part 4) are sometimes called "psychobiotics."[4] Various other psychiatric conditions such as autism, schizophrenia, bipolar disorder, or obsessive-compulsive disorder, all show links to gut microbiota to a larger or smaller extent. Further experiments in this area will determine whether the observed gut dysbiosis in these disorders are consequences of poor diet, medication, or infections, or are direct contributors. This will guide future therapeutic approaches.[5]

Another field of research on the microbial gut–brain axis is neurodegenerative diseases and injuries, such as Parkinson's disease (PD), Alzheimer's disease (AD), stroke, epilepsy, ALS, Huntington's disease, and others. Constipation is one of the PD symptoms, starting much earlier than the motoric symptoms (such as tremors). Abnormal aggregations of a protein called alpha-synuclein in the brain are a typical sign of PD and interestingly, have been also observed in the gut branches of the vagus nerve in the early phases of PD. There is an ongoing debate about whether these protein aggregations could be transported to the brain via the vagus and, if and how gut microbes influence their formation. There is also a lot of research about the possible roles of pathogenic microbes (including viruses) in the progression of AD. As previously mentioned, dysbiosis with higher or lower levels of specific microbes is often observed but more studies are needed to show clear links to the pathology of each disease.

Metabolic Diseases: Sedentary Life isn't All Cracked Up To Be

Just as your laptop or smartphone needs electricity to work, your brain needs only two things: glucose and oxygen. As the main energy source, glucose is constantly monitored by the body and it must be always kept within a narrow range (around 80–120 mg/l). If our brain senses too low glucose, we feel hungry. If the food doesn't arrive, the body activates reserves of sugars from the liver and, if that is not enough, also from our fat reserves. On the other hand, after a meal (or a snack) when glucose rises in the blood, the pancreatic cells in our bodies release the hormone insulin, signaling our cells to absorb excess glucose and, within a short time, glucose levels return to normal. However, the regulation of feelings of hunger and satiety is a more complex issue. For example, chemicals secreted by the above-mentioned EC and EEC cells in the gut wall can regulate insulin production and its release from the pancreas or via the blood system or enteric nervous system and vagus nerve, sending signals directly to the brain. Experiments in mice have shown that molecules produced by gut microbes (e.g. SCFA, bile acids, LPS) can regulate secretion by EC and EEC cells, thus indirectly signaling to the brain and regulating glucose levels and appetite. Some microbes such as lactobacilli or bifidobacteria, can even directly produce human neurotransmitters[8].[6]

Obesity is a metabolic disease hitting global epidemic proportions during the last decades. According to the study called "Health Effects of Overweight and Obesity in 195 Countries over 25 Years" (2017), around 10 percent of all humans can be characterized as obese, that is more than 600 million adults and more than 100 million children in 196 countries.[7] In the United States alone, around 43 percent of the population is obese. Obesity is characterized by extreme accumulation of body fat, which can lead to other metabolic diseases such as type 2 (T2D) diabetes, cardio-metabolic diseases, kidney, liver, and other organ failures. Obesity is caused by a combination of lack of physical activity, highly caloric food, genetic, and environmental factors. Studies on mice, however, have taught us that the gut microbiome also plays an important role in obesity pathology. Namely, by transferring the gut microbiome from an obese to a lean (GF) mouse, scientists could make it obese.[8] Further studies in animals and humans have shown that the observed metabolic effects of the gut microbiome are on multiple levels:

a) the above-mentioned gut–brain axis and the satiety hormones;
b) connections of the microbiome with the immune system, in particular, the development of the immune system in children and the observed chronic low-grade inflammation in obese people, linked with the integrity of the gut wall;
c) influence of the gut microbes on the metabolism of nutrients (for example, by harvesting energy from non-digestible food) and lipid metabolism.[9]

Diabetes is another global metabolic disease, with more than 9 percent of the world population affected in 2019. There are two types of diabetes: Type 1 (T1D) in which the blood sugar spikes because insulin-producing cells of the pancreas are destroyed, and T2D, in which body cells don't react to insulin properly (insulin resistance) and/or less insulin is produced by the pancreas. The connection between T1D and the microbiome is still debated, but there is more evidence for the role of gut microbes in T2D pathology. Similar to obesity, observed changes include gut dysbiosis (for example higher Firmicutes/Proteobacteria and Bacteroidetes ratio and lower Akker-mannsia), leaky gut wall, and increased inflammation-markers. Many of these microbial markers are observed already in the pre-diabetic stages of T2D.[10]

Substantial changes in gut microbiomes and specific microbial metabolites have been also observed in cardio-metabolic diseases (such as atherosclerosis), liver diseases (Non-Alcoholic Fat Liver Disease or NAFLD), and malnutrition.[11] Future therapeutic approaches to these diseases include dietary intervention, probiotic and others which we will discuss in the part.

Finally, Let's Listen to Our Gut

We have read about IBD in Chapter 7. Let's understand it as one of the conditions.

IBD is one of the chronic inflammatory diseases of the gastrointestinal tract (GI tract) which is portrayed by intermittent episodes of inflammation. Depending upon the disease location and depth of involvement in the GI tract, these inflammations can be divided into two types of intestinal disease (for which the cause is mostly unknown), known as *Ulcerative colitis* (UC) and *Crohn's disease* (CD)[12]. Unfortunately, causes of both are mostly unknown.

UC is characterized by continuous ascending inflammation initiating in the end part of the large intestine (rectum) and extending in the colon (major part of the large intestine) with periods of improvement and worsening of the symptoms (relapse). Inflammation in UC, However, inflammation causes superficial damage to the bowel wall as it is typically limited to the mucosa, slimy layer located at the colonic surface. On average, 50 percent of the diagnosed UC patients suffer from relapses over time relapse[15,16,13] and are prone to develop colon cancer later in life. *Pouchitis*, is a most frequent complication of UC, developed after surgical removal of inflamed colon. In this treatment, after removal of colon, end part of the small gut (ileum) can be surgically joined with rectum, forming a pouch (a pocket-like structure). However, after some time inflammation can develop even within the ileal pouch. Factors contributing to pouchitis and its pathogenesis are largely unknown.

In contrast, CD is characterized by intestinal lesions (areas with abnormal tissue) anywhere in the GI tract. The inflammation in CD is worsening over time and affects whole gut tissue, eventually leading to chronic abdominal cramping, persistent diarrhea, constipation, and injuries in the anal region.[14] Also, severity in CD is much higher as compared to UC, because inflammation in CD is not superficial and it is continuous. Intestinal complications of CD are very common and almost half of all patients show narrowing or abnormal opening of the bowel within 10 years after diagnosis. Also, bowel damage at the time of diagnosis and surgery requirement are commonly seen events from several studies. Around 21–47 percent CD patients show systemic and other symptoms beyond gut, such as arthritis, iron deficiency, anemia creeping fat, and osteoporosis, which all increases risk of hospitalization. Another manifestation of CD is *creeping fat*, a process by which adipose tissue outside the gut migrates towards intestinal lesions, narrowing the bowel.[15]

The role of gut microbiome in IBD is an emerging area of research. The factors that regulate the abnormal immune responses in UC and CD, leading to intestinal inflammation (along with the other manifestations beyond gut) might be genetic, environmental but also *microbial*. Gut microbes were even suspected to be one of the potential infectious agents although the process of causation hasn't been yet proven.

Several studies have explored microbial differences (based on the presence/absence of microbes and how many times a microbe is present) along the length of the GI tract and their associations with IBD pathogenesis[16]. Major intestinal vulnerabilities that contribute to IBD and the role of microbial communities in aggravating or preventing the onset of disease have been reported. Though bacterial components of microbial communities have been studied a lot, recent studies have shown the impact of other microbes such as viruses and fungi in the progression of IBD.[17]

Changes in the Composition and Function of Gut Microbial Communities Associated with Active IBD

There are several microbial features associated with patients suffering from UC and CD. For instance, 1) lower microbial diversity,[18] 2) higher abundance of Enterobacteria, Proteobacteria, *Escherichia coli*, *Ruminococcus gnavus*, Bacteroidetes in CD and/or UC patients,[19] 3) lower abundance of Clostridia, *Bifidobacterium*, *Lactobacillus*, *Faecalibacterium prausnitzii*, *Alistipes putredinis*, *Roseburia hominis* in CD and/or UC patients.[20] Similarly, several microbial functional changes are also associated with IBD for example, 1) higher levels of *N*-acylethanolamines, a class of endogenously produced signaling lipids, lower levels of pathways involved in the polysaccharide degradation, proteinogenic amino acid degradation, and lower levels of genes associated with butanoate and propanoate metabolism, and biosynthesis of amino acids.[21] At metabolites level, lower levels of fecal short-chain fatty acids (mainly produced by the fermentation of complex carbohydrates), such as butyrate and acetate, along with reduced levels of methylamine and trimethylamine were also reported in Crohn's disease.[22]

Taken together, reports have suggested drastic changes in the microbial and functional diversity and abundance of fecal and mucosa-associated bacterial composition along the GI tract [23].

Tissue samples (biopsy) are typically obtained after surgical operations and therefore, fecal samples are the most commonly used non-invasive method to detect which microbes are living in the intestinal tract. It is crucial to understand the sample type before accessing the microbiome because in biopsies microbial presence might be different from fecal samples. In the case of biopsies, it is also important to know the sample site from where the samples were collected (such as the ascending colon, descending colon, ileum, or rectum) because each sampling site, after all, has a variable microbiome. However, there are many challenges in studying the contribution of individual microbial communities toward the progression of IBD. For example, the fecal microbial composition contains mostly the luminal component (microbes present in the bowel which can flush out with the feces) and may therefore not accurately reflect the bacterial species enriched/depleted in the mucosal epithelium of the GI tract. To understand the actual drivers of disease, microbial profiling needs to be done at the site of inflammation, such as the proximal colon for UC and in the ileum for CD. All "omics" approaches described in the chapter about microbiome analysis (16S rRNA gene sequencing, shotgun metagenomics, metatranscriptomics, metaproteomics, and metabolomics) can be used to understand the compositional, functional, and metabolic changes in the microbial communities at the species and strain levels.

Bacterial components and their functions are most widely studied to understand their probable roles in IBD. However, there are other poorly investigated non-bacterial components of the gut microbiome that may also be relevant. One such component is the mycobiome—composition of fungal communities residing in the gut—which plays an important role in regulating the host immune systems through the innate immune receptor, Dectin-1.[24] Fungal community analysis from multiple studies using mucosal and fecal samples showed increased abundance and associations of *Candida albicans, Aspergillus clavatus, Candida neoformans, Saccharomyces cerevisiae, Clavispora lusitaniae, Cyberlindnera jadinii,* and *Kluyveromyces marxianus* species in CD patients.[25]

Gut Infection: A Case of *Clostridum difficile*

Clostridium difficile is a bacterium that can act as a pathogen in the gut and is one of the causes of a gut infection. This pathogen is the most frequent complication resulting out of antibiotic therapy that affects thousands of people every year worldwide.[26] Often perfectly healthy people have *C. difficile* in their gut which, if left undisturbed, coexists peacefully with other members of the microbial gut community. Similar to some other bacterial species, *C. difficile* can survive harsh external conditions by thickening its cell walls and forming so-called spores, which are dormant cells that can survive long periods without nutrients and are resistant to many antibiotics and antiseptic chemicals. However when antibiotic therapy causes depletion of other gut bacteria, *C. difficile* gets the opportunity to quickly multiply by using excess gut nutrients which would be normally used by other bacteria and becomes the dominant species. This is how *C. difficile* infection (CDI) occurs, typically manifesting as mild to severe diarrhea with fever, which in the majority of cases is successfully treated by antibiotics. However, in about 20–30 percent of the patients, infection will come back in a few weeks and if these patients are treated with antibiotics again, chances of getting the next round of CDI are even higher, entering a vicious cycle of a life-threatening condition called recurrent CDI (rCDI).[27] Ironically, the condition caused by antibiotics is treated again with antibiotics. Microbiome transplantation seems a promising option against rCDI, which we will discuss in the part about microbiome-based therapies.

Coeliac Disease

On the inner surface of the intestines (epithelium) lies small finger-like protrusions called "villi." They increase the surface of the intestines and enable the efficient absorption of nutrients. Coeliac disease is caused when the small intestine's immune cells start attacking their own body's cells, destroying villi due to an error in the immune system (as in other autoimmune diseases). Intolerance to the protein gluten (found in wheat, barley, and rye) is one of the typical symptoms of the disease. Except for genetic factors, other factors triggering Coeliac disease are unknown. Studies have shown that microbial diversity, intestinal infection in early life, and the presence of specific bacteria could play a role in the pathogenesis and severity of Coeliac disease. Probiotics or bacterial strains capable of degrading gluten have been proposed as possible therapeutic approaches.[28] We will discuss these approaches in other sections of the book.

CHAPTER 9

SKIN, ORAL AND RESPIRATORY CONDITIONS ONE MUST KNOW!

Skin Conditions

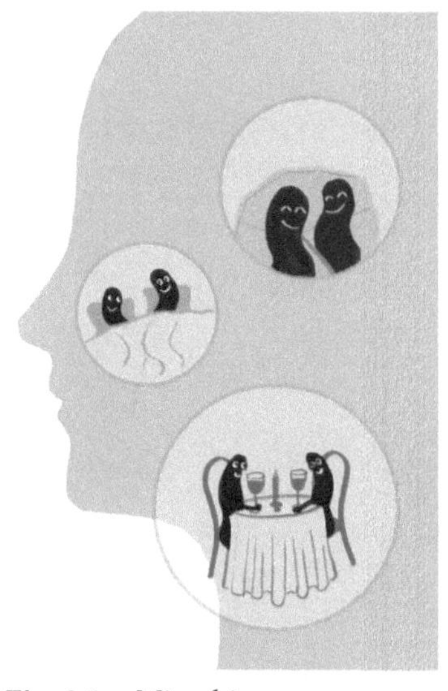

Fig. 9.1 Microbiomes are present all over human skin

THE beauty and cosmetic market is flooded with acne-treating lotions and potions. Instagram influencers are promoting various skin brands' products by narrating their own stories of clearing breakouts. A tired teenager would try anything to help their skin breakouts but how many times do these products actually help? Do you know that if your breakouts aren't getting any better that means the product you are using is probably killing beneficial bacteria on your skin while stimulating the growth of the potentially pathogenic ones? Or that your nutrition may indirectly influence your skin microbiome by influencing your gut microbiome? Or that your mood can influence your skin microbiome?

Let's try to understand how microbiomes affect our skin health.

It might sound paradoxical, but our skin and our gut have similarities:

a) Both are our barriers to the outside world, although common sense tells us that while the gut is "inside" our bodies, its content, from mouth to anus, is "outside" the body.

b) Both are covered by a lining of cells (epithelium), preventing unwanted molecules to penetrate through. The difference however is that the gut epithelium is covered by a thick layer of slime (mucus) and the skin, the outermost layer (epidermis), by a hard cover made of a protein called keratin (also including dead skin cells). Additional skin protection is provided by its light acidity (pH 4.7–5.75) and a layer of fat (sebum) produced by special skin glands (sebaceous glands).

c) Both have a dense network of blood vessels, nerves, and immune cells.

d) Both have their own microbiomes.[1]

Often the gut conditions, such as the previously mentioned inflammatory bowel disease, have skin manifestations in the form of redness, skin ulcers, and other abnormal tissue changes.[2] As mentioned in the previous chapter, gut microbes (directly), and specialized gut cells (upon stimulation by the gut microbes) produce hormones, some of which enter the blood, affecting the skin and skin microbiome. This can be indirectly triggered through the gut–brain axis, which could explain skin reactions to stress or anxiety. Because of these close connections between the skin and the gut through the immune and nervous systems, the term "gut–skin-axis" is often used.[3]

By virtue of the connection of the skin with the gut–brain axis and the presence of specific skin microbiota, it is possible to classify skin diseases into two main groups:

1. The first group has all the pathologies caused by altered functioning of the immune system (atopic dermatitis, psoriasis, urticaria, lupus, lichen), and these will inevitably be associated with alterations of the intestinal microbiota (although there are usually changes in the composition of the skin microbiota, too).
2. The second group includes infections and is treated as such (acne, seborrheic dermatitis, rosacea, pityriasis versicolor). These are associated with alterations of the skin microbiota and must, from now on, be considered microbial skin dysbiosis.

There can also be a third group that could include two autoimmune diseases (alopecia areata and vitiligo) which likely derive from an alteration of the intestinal microbiota but which probably occur in areas where there is also an alteration of the skin microbiota.

In the next few lines, we will discuss a few of the skin diseases from each of these groups.

In Chapter 1, we mentioned that different areas of our skin have different microbiomes. Dry areas of our skin, such as our hands or arms, tend to have a higher diversity of microbes than, for example, moist areas such as our armpits. In various skin conditions, the structure of these microbial communities is changed, causing microbial dysbiosis.

Most of us have probably experienced symptoms like skin redness, dryness, swelling, or itchiness. In more serious cases, these could be symptoms of a condition called **atopic dermatitis** (AD), also known as atopic eczema. The exact cause of AD is not known. Genetic factors and the immune system (affected areas are inflamed) most likely play a role. AD in young children can be severe, covering the whole body. AD patients are also prone to allergies and asthma, which is another hint of a connection to the immune system. AD patients have elevated levels of the bacterium *Staphylococcus aureus*, typically found in wounds and skin infections. On the other hand, there are fewer bacteria of some other types (such as *Cutibacterium, Streptococcus, Acinetobacter, Corynebacterium, Prevotella*).[4]

Pimples, papules, pustules, whiteheads, and blackheads are something teenagers and young adults are scared and ashamed of. In medical jargon, they all have one common name: **acne vulgaris**. Unfortunately, more than eighty percent of adolescents and young adults are affected by this condition.[5] Typically, it happens on the oily skin parts when the pores around the tiny hairs get blocked by the skin oil and the dead skin cells, causing inflammation. Adolescents are considered to be the most affected group due to the excess oil production by the skin glands (caused by hormonal changes in puberty). Until now *Cutibacterium acnes* has always been identified as the causative agent of acne, but it is found both in patients and in healthy individuals. We now know that *C. acnes* are not all the same: analysis of genes from the skin microbiome samples (metagenomic analysis, explained in Chapter 2) has shown that while the relative abundances of *C. acnes* are similar, the structures of the strain population can differ significantly. Some strains are highly associated with acne and other strains are more abundant in healthy skin. Also, the balance between *C. acnes*, *Streptococcus epidermidis*, and *Staphylococcus aureus* seems (all typical bacteria of the normal skin), seems to be important for acne formation.[6]

Interestingly, acne is completely absent in the indigenous (hunter-gatherer) human population, suggesting links with the diet (in particular Western-style diet) and the gut microbiome.[7]

Psoriasis and **rosacea** are two other serious skin inflammatory diseases. **Psoriasis** is characterized by smaller or bigger areas of abnormal skin (plaques or pustules), which are differently colored (e.g. red or purple), dry, and itchy. It is caused by a combination of environmental and genetic factors, but gut dysbiosis (and therefore the immune system component) is also typical.[8] Specific bacterial species, such as staphylococci are found to be dominant around the affected areas.[9] In **rosacea**, skin blood vessels are affected by inflammation, causing smaller or larger areas of the face to become red. Increased densities of normal skin mite *Demodex folliculorum* (mentioned in Chapter 1), as well as several other usual skin bacteria (such as *Staphylococcus epidermidis*) are found near the affected skin areas but the exact role of these microbes is yet to be clarified.[10]

Can Our Scalp be an Affected Area?

Dandruff, small white flakes falling from your hair on your dark cloth can be very annoying. Again, microbiome analysis showed higher levels of normal skin fungus Malassezia; not common Malassezia species, but some that are not yet characterized.[11] Bacterial composition is also different: in people, without dandruff, the Propionibacterium make up 71 percent of the flora and the staphylococci 26 percent while in the producers of dandruff the balances are different, with the Propionibacterium at 50 percent and the staphylococci at 44 percent.[12]

The same discourse applies to seborrheic dermatitis, larger skin flakes falling off the scalp (but also other skin areas such as eyebrow, nose, ear, etc.) for which Malassezia was also previously considered responsible. Today, however, we know that seborrheic dermatitis is a multi-pathogenic disease, caused by the dysbiosis of both fungi and bacteria.

Hair loss in men (known as androgenic alopecia) is typical for many men of a certain age. It is basically micro-inflammation of the hair follicle with genetic and hormonal causes though differences in microbiomes of the hair follicles have been found between men with and without hair loss.[13] The more serious hair-loss condition is the autoimmune disease alopecia areata (AA). It occurs both in men and women and hair is lost only in certain areas of the head, whole head, or whole body. Reasons for it are unknown, but the immune component (including gut microbiota) and psychological stress probably play a role. Certain fungal species were associated with AA and two cases of hair regrowth after fecal microbiome transplant (see the chapter on therapeutical applications) suggest a probable role of the gut microbiome.[14]

Can Microbiomes Make Our Skin Younger?

Besides gut–skin axis and specific body area, aging is an important factor affecting the composition of the skin microbiome. Although previous studies identified changes in the makeup of the skin microbiome related to aging, researchers had yet to fully understand the mechanisms behind these changes. Indeed, skin aging is a normal and unavoidable process characterized by structural and functional changes in skin cells, as a result of biological age, as well as external factors (e.g. exposure to ultraviolet radiation, toxins, and poor nutrition).[15] Skin aging is also affected by decreasing epidermal thickness and water content, fat emulsion, lipid content, and changes in amino acid composition.[16] Previous studies highlighted other fundamental intrinsic human variables that influence the density and diversity of microbes present in various host skin areas. For example, some face skin characteristics, such as hydration, are known to vary across individuals and even between various parts of the skin within one individual. But, these skin features and their interplay with microbial flora are not fully understood. We know that many of the current therapies for skin conditions, such as antibiotics or corticosteroids, are not efficient or even more damaging, due to the disturbance of the natural microbial balance. Therefore, new, microbiome-based therapies are desperately needed. We will discuss more about probiotics and postbiotics later in Part IV of this book. Companies such as AOBiome, Matrysis, SkinBioTherapeutics, Dermabiont, Evelo, and others are currently developing microbiome-based therapies for many inflammatory skin conditions, but also for infections and wound healing.

Many questions remain open: which factors are critical for damage to the skin barrier preceding a disease (e.g. UV light, externally applied chemicals, etc.)? What are the roles of individual skin microbes (or their metabolites) in various skin diseases? How does the interplay between the gut microbiome, immune system, and skin exactly work?

We hope that the ongoing efforts of many researchers will help us to find answers to these questions in the near future.

Oral Conditions

The force of a human bite is as high as 1000 Newtons (N). Under normal conditions, the weight of one kilogram exerts 10 N force on a surface. This means when we bite a peanut, our teeth presses a weight of one hundred kilograms on it. Besides sea otters, bears, and pigs, humans are among few mammal species having such a powerful tool in their mouths. For this, we can largely thank the amazing material called enamel, covering the surface of our teeth.[8] Despite its strength, tiny microorganisms in our mouth consume sugar and produce acid that gradually cracks the enamel. Though small initially, these damages over a longer period of time become dental cavities also known as dental caries.

Another common oral disease is gum disease, also known as periodontal disease or periodontitis. It is an inflammation of the gums mostly caused by bacteria in the tissue surrounding the teeth and, if not treated, it can lead to loosening and loss of teeth. A milder form of gum inflammation (which typically precedes gum disease) is called gingivitis.

For decades since the 1950s, *Streptococcus mutans* was a bacterium considered the main causative agent of caries. Another bacterium, *Porphyromonas gingivalis*, was linked to gum disease.[9] With the advances in microbiological and sequencing methods, it became clearer that the situation in our mouths is much more complex. Recent studies have shown that more than 370 bacterial species can be potential biomarkers for caries, among which are acid-producing streptococci and lactobacilli, including many others. Among the highly abundant species, *Streptococcus mutans* consisted of only 1.2 percent. Bacterial species such as *Tannerella forsythia*, *Treponema denticola*, and also many others, previously uncultivated, have been found around the gum sites affected by periodontic disease.[17] The exact roles of these species, as well as other microbes (such as oral fungi and viruses), in the genesis and progression of diseases of teeth, gums, and oral mucosa and oral cancers are yet to be determined.

In the literature, oral microbiomes have been often associated with other, systemic health conditions. Examples include cardiovascular diseases, gastrointestinal cancers (like pancreatic), liver cirrhosis, irritable bowel disease, Alzheimer's disease, and others.

Oral bacterial communities are typically organized in so-called biofilms, complex structures of multiple layers of bacteria, embedded in an organic matrix they produce. On the teeth surfaces, these biofilms are called dental plaque and their composition is specific for each individual, depending on many external factors such as diet, smoking, other existing diseases (such as diabetes), stress, or status of the immune system.[18] Brushing and flossing to remove dental plaque are the best preventive ways against oral diseases. However, the application of broad-range antibacterial mouthwashes, such as chlorhexidine (CHX), considered for a long time as a standard concept of oral hygiene, has been shown to reduce overall bacterial diversity, increasing acidity (therefore creating caries-causing conditions) and blood pressure. A newer concept of anti-caries strategy is the introduction of beneficial (probiotic) bacteria which can reduce oral acidity and the level of caries-causing species.[19]

What Happens When We Breathe In

> *"Sometimes, all I need is the air that I breathe and to love you."*
>
> —Song by The Hollies

"Aeros" in Old Greek. "Life energy" (*prana*) in Sanskrit. "Spirit that is everywhere" (*vozduh*) in several Slavic languages. Around seven thousand liters of it goes in and out of our lungs daily. It travels through our mouth and nose, all the channels and cavities in our head, down through the throat, and into our lungs, where finally it exchanges gases with our blood. Anatomically, our airways are divided into upper and lower parts.

Microbiomes of the upper airways seem to be important for inflammatory conditions such as chronic respiratory sinusitis, but also the pathology of other lung diseases, such as cystic fibrosis (CF). Links to neurological conditions, such as Parkinson's disease (PD) or Alzheimer's disease (AD), and multiple sclerosis (MS) have been also suggested.[20] The influence of microbiomes on the sense of smell (olfactory receptors) is an active topic of research. The loss of smell has been reported as one of the early symptoms of PD and AD and, as many of us recently learned, of COVID-19.[21]

Lower airways, including the lungs, get their microbes from the upper airways. Until recently, people believed that lower airways are sterile. Sampling by medical examination techniques such as bronchoalveolar lavage (BAL), followed by sequencing, have uncovered disruptions in lung microbiome (dysbiosis) in lung conditions such as chronic obstructive pulmonary disease (COPD), asthma, lung cancer, COVID-19, and others.[22] Similar to other microbiomes, researchers are trying to define microbes that can be used for the diagnosis, prevention, or prognosis of these diseases. In general, in a healthy state, the lung microbiome has low microbial density but high diversity. In a diseased state, it is the opposite; diversity decreases but the overall density of microbes is higher[23]

Gut–lung axis is also an important field of research. Diet, use of antibiotics, or other external factors can change our gut microbiota. As we will see in Part 4, metabolites produced by the gut microbes (such as short chain fatty acids) influence immune response in the lungs. However, this communication seems to be bidirectional since patients with COPD or CF often experience gut symptoms (dysbiosis)[24]

CHAPTER 10

HOW VAGINAL AND NEWBORN MICROBIOME INFLUENCES HEALTH

Vaginal Health and How to Keep it Balanced

THERE is increasing evidence that genital tract health is strongly influenced by the interplay between the microorganisms residing in the reproductive system and the host.

Would you believe that a woman's vaginal microbiome plays an important role in her sexual and reproductive health? There are multiple mechanisms linking the vaginal microbiome composition and function with poor health outcomes. As shortly described in Chapter 1, the microbiome in the female reproductive system is different from the vagina to the cervix and uterus. The microbiome of the vagina is the most studied part of the female reproductive system since collecting samples from the vagina is less invasive compared to collecting samples from other areas of the reproductive system. Here's how it happens:

Gynecologists sometimes collect samples from the vagina during yearly check-ups for a quick assessment of the vagina's health. This method is called a vaginal wet mount test or vaginal smear and is often performed if there is an indication of a vaginal infection. So, how is the test conducted? The doctor collects samples from the vaginal wall using a swab. The sample collected is smeared on a microscope slide and mixed with saline solution and then visualized under the microscope. This quick and easy method allows doctors to determine what type of bacteria are present in the vagina based on their shape. The presence of rod-shaped cells, similar to small sticks, on the slide indicates that the majority of bacteria are *Lactobacillus*.

How to Determine the Health of the Vagina?

Vaginas colonized mainly by bacteria of the *Lactobacillus* group, especially *Lactobacillus crispatus*, are associated with good health. A low diverse vaginal microbiome and a low pH of around 4-4,5 are indicators of a healthy vagina. The vaginal microbes coexist with the human host in a mutualistic relationship, in which the lactobacilli offer protection against pathogens and the host provides nutrients for their growth, therefore both parties involved benefit from this relationship.

Although *Lactobacillus*-dominated vaginal microbiome has been associated with a healthy vaginal microbiome, not all *Lactobacillus* species are the same, and not all women's vaginal microbiota contains a majority of the bacteria from the *Lactobacillus* group. Around 80–89 percent of Asian and Caucasian women have a *Lactobacillus*-dominated vaginal microbiome, while in women of African and Hispanic ancestry only 59–62 percent of women have this type of vaginal microbiome.[1] Depending on the majority of microbial species present in the vagina, scientists have classified the vaginal microbiome into 5 different types, known as community state types (CSTs). Four of these communities are characterized by an increased presence of 4 different *Lactobacillus* species, namely *L. crispatus* (CST I), *Lactobacillus gasseri* (CST II), *Lactobacillus iners* (CST III), and *Lactobacillus jensenii*

(CST V). A CST IV vaginal microbiome has reduced numbers of *Lactobacillus* bacteria and increased abundance of other bacteria, such as *Gardnerella vaginalis, Prevotella, Streptococcus, Atopobium,* and others. Generally, the presence of a polymicrobial community such as the CST IV is often associated with a less healthy vaginal microbiome and an increased risk of vaginal infections and other associated vaginal diseases.

The Vaginal Microbiome is Dynamic and Changes Under the Influence of Different Factors

Similar to other human microbiomes, the vaginal microbiome is not static, but rather dynamic and changes over time. It can shift across years; women have a different vaginal microbiome before their first period compared to the time when they are of reproductive age and it changes again during pregnancy and even after menopause.[2] Moreover, day-to-day behavior can affect the vaginal microbiome and lead to compositional changes. For example, taking medication, especially antibiotics and birth control, smoking, use of vaginal products, vaginal douching, sexual partners, stress, smoking, and poor hygiene are just a few of the factors that can lead to shifts in the vaginal microbiome composition toward an unstable, dysbiotic state.[3.]

Another factor that strongly influences the vaginal microbiome is female hormones, especially estrogen. Studies have shown that as soon as the reproductive age of a woman begins, the rise in estrogen level promotes changes in the vaginal mucosa leading to increased content of glycogen. Glycogen is a multibranched complex sugar formed of many glucose molecules which is further transformed by the human enzymes into metabolites that act as food for bacteria. *Lactobacillus* species use these glycogen metabolites to generate energy and, in this process, lactic acid is produced that leads to a reduction of pH in the vaginal environment, thus protecting against pathogenic bacteria, as many of these "bad" bacteria cannot grow at low pH values.[4] Besides lactic acid, *Lactobacillus* species can produce other anti-bacterial substances called bacteriocins, which are natural antibiotics that inhibit the growth of harmful bacteria.

Another mechanism by which *Lactobacillus* can protect against vaginal infections is to attach to vaginal epithelial cells and form a protective layer thus outcompeting other bacteria for the same space. And last, they can modulate the immune system and keep inflammation down in the genital tract. However, not all *Lactobacillus* species offer the same protection. The presence of *L. crispatus* in the vagina is always associated with a healthy vaginal microbiome, while *L. iners* is more associated with a vaginal microbiome prone to infection. The reason is that *L. iners* produces only one form of lactic acid, named L-lactic acid which is less effective against pathogens than the other form, D-lactic acid. Furthermore, *L. iners* is more dependent on the host for additional resources, thus if the resources for its growth are not present, *L. iners* can be outcompeted by other bacteria, which are less protective. Sometimes, *L. iners* acts as a shapeshifter. In the presence of other *Lactobacillus* species, it has either a neutral or protective role, but in the company of other diverse bacteria it can cause symptoms like itching and unusual discharge.[5.]

Dysbiosis in the Vaginal Microbiome Can Lead to Vaginal Infections

Bacterial vaginosis is the most widespread vaginal infection among women of reproductive age and it affects more than 30 percent of women worldwide. This disease is characterized by a strong loss of *Lactobacillus* species and an increase in the number of facultative or obligate anaerobic bacteria such as *Gardnerella*, *Prevotella*, *Atopobium*, *Ureaplasma*, *Mycoplasma*, and others. The cause of bacterial vaginosis is not fully understood. Sometimes external factors and a woman's behavior can cause changes in the vaginal environment which may lead to disbalance in the vaginal microbiome, thus triggering the beginning of an infection. The microbes causing the bacterial vaginosis form biofilms on the vaginal epithelium and through their toxic action healthy cells of the vagina are killed and inflammation is triggered. This cascade of events often leads to symptoms that are experienced by women such as unusual milk-like vaginal discharge that has a strong fishy odor. Bacterial vaginosis doesn't always manifest symptoms in all women. Some women have the infection without any symptoms[6.]

Now, if you wonder what are biofilms? As previously explained in the chapter about oral microbiomes, biofilms are complex conglomerations of different microorganisms that stick together and are kept together by slimy substances. Biofilms are sometimes referred to as "cities of microorganisms." The problem with biofilms and especially biofilms formed by pathogenic bacteria is that the microbes living in these conglomerations are hard to reach and sometimes treatments do not work properly. Often treatment of bacterial vaginosis will help with reducing the symptoms but without fully removing the cause. This is one of the reasons why bacterial vaginosis is hard to treat and often women who had this disease, might experience a relapse after some months.[7]

Some unusual smelly discharge may not sound that bad, but untreated bacterial vaginosis can cause serious problems. Pregnant women who have bacterial vaginosis are at higher risk to give birth prematurely, which is often accompanied by increased mortality of preterm babies and can experience late miscarriage, amniotic fluid infections, and other complications. In non-pregnant women, bacterial vaginosis increases the risk of urinary tract infections and other pelvic diseases, including cervical cancer. Moreover, bacterial vaginosis is also associated with an increased risk of acquiring sexually transmitted diseases.[8.]

Current therapies for bacterial vaginosis include the use of antibiotics with a broad activity that can target the polymicrobial infection and the use of probiotics that can help in restoring the healthy vaginal microbiome. These therapies have not always been successful in fully treating bacterial vaginosis, that is why new therapeutic strategies are being developed such as novel compounds that can disrupt the biofilm and kill the culprit bacteria, microbial live therapeutics based on *L. crispatus* strains, and even vaginal microbiota transplant from healthy women.[9]

Is Infertility Linked to the Vaginal Microbiome Composition?

Statistics show that up to 10 percent of women struggle with infertility,[10] and in many cases, the cause of infertility remains unexplained. Scientific research has looked at possible correlations between vaginal microbiome composition and infertility as well as the success of in vitro fertilization (IVF). Although some observational studies indicate a possible connection between vaginal dysbiosis, infertility, and a low chance of IVF success, most of the data remains conflicting. The microbiome composition of other areas of the reproductive tract may be important for IVF success.[11] For example, scientists looked at the endometrium microbiome of infertile women who underwent IVF and discovered that women who had an increased number of *Lactobacillus* strains in their endometrial microbiome showed higher rates of implantation and live birth rate.[12] Up to now, there is no direct link between the vaginal microbiome and infertility, although bacterial vaginosis is known to cause problems both in non-pregnant and pregnant women, more data is needed to understand the role of the vaginal microbiome and the microbiome in other areas of the reproductive tract in women's fertility.

Keeping a healthy vaginal microbiome

Maintaining a healthy lifestyle will improve the health of the microbiome as well. Practicing good behaviors by eating nutritious food, exercising regularly, minimizing stress, and maintaining general good hygiene are essential for overall well-being and for supporting a balanced microbiome.

When it comes to the vaginal microbiome, keeping tabs on its composition through available vaginal health tests or simply by occasionally checking at home the pH values of the vagina, can help women to identify any imbalances early on and act to promote a protective microbiome.

Infant Microbiome in Health and Disease

The microbiome development in infants is a journey toward a stable healthy microbiome. The first 1,000 days after birth are considered highly important for the growth and development of infants. Perturbations that occur within this critical window can impair the healthy development and growth of infants and their microbiome.[13]

The journey starts in the mother's womb. As the fetus is developing it meets the microorganisms for the first time. Although there is an ongoing debate if infants acquire any microbiomes when they are in the womb, many studies have shown evidence that infants are not born sterile.[14] Birth is an important event for the development of a healthy microbiome. Infants who are born vaginally, while passing through the birth canal come in contact with billions of microbes from the mother who quickly colonize their skin and reach the colon through ingestion starting a new life there. Infants that are born through cesarean section, also known as "C-section," miss this important event. The first microbes that C-section-born infants come in contact with are microbes from the environment and the skin. These microbes can also form the first colonies in the infant's gut.[15] There have been many studies trying to elucidate the importance of birth mode on the development of a healthy microbiome. Although C-section infants are at higher risk of developing certain diseases later in life, it is not entirely clear whether such risk is mainly linked to being born C-section or to other unfavorable events that can happen in the first 1,000 days of a newborn's life. Two other events that are equally important for the development of a healthy gut microbiome, are breastfeeding and the use of antibiotics.

You've probably heard the phrase "you are what you eat." It also holds true for the microbiome. Diet has a huge influence on gut microbiome composition and function, so what we eat will shape the microbiome. For infants, the food they receive in the first months of life is even more important that the dietary changes adults experience throughout their life. Hence health organizations recommend that infants should be breastfed at least during the first 6 months of life and continue to do so if the mother can for some more months.[16.] Of course, introducing solid foods is also an important event, but let's start with the first 6 months of life.

For an infant's wholesome growth and development, breast milk contains all the nutrients. Besides these nutrients, a mother's milk contains nonessential nutrients that are not digested by infants, the so-called human milk oligosaccharides (HMOs).[17]These non-digestible oligosaccharides, which are nothing more than sugars, are not nutrients for the infant but are rather nourishing specific groups of gut bacteria, such as *Bifidobacterium* and *Bacteroides*. Moreover, mother's milk also contains microorganisms that are passed to infants and are important for a healthy seeding of microbiomes.[18] The development of a healthy microbiome is crucially important for the development of the immune system. During the early development of infants, the microbiome will communicate with the host through the metabolites it produces and other mechanisms. It teaches the immune system how to distinguish between friends and foes. When the immune system recognizes a microbe as a foe, a cascade of events will be triggered that is often accompanied by inflammation which can lead to damage to epithelial cells in the gut and further contribute to the development of diseases

Infants who are fed formula do not get these beneficial microbes from their food and their good microorganisms will not obtain the necessary nutrients needed to grow and outcompete other bacteria, which are less favorable for early gut microbiome development.[19] Nowadays, companies try to formulate formula milk as similar as possible to the mother's milk. There are more and more baby formulas available that contain either probiotics or human oligosaccharides besides other nutrients. Developing a formula that fully mimics the breastmilk composition is not possible, as breastmilk contains various nutrients that are unique to each mother and infant. Furthermore, there are more than 200 different human oligosaccharides, and each mother produces different combinations of HMOs that are present in the milk and transferred to the infants during breastfeeding. It is important to note that the mother's behavior will influence the breastmilk composition and microbiome, therefore a healthy diet and lifestyle and limiting antibiotic use during the breastfeeding period are important.[20] One study in Canada has shown that pumped breastmilk does not have the same microbial composition as the milk directly from the breast, and depending on how the pumped milk is stored and handled, there is the possibility that enrichment in pathogenic bacteria may occur, that is why whenever possible mothers should breastfeed their infants.

After the first 6 months, it is recommended that different solid and liquid foods should be included gradually in an infant's diet.[21] This process is known as weaning, switching an infant's diet from breastfeeding or formula feeding to solid and liquid foods. This process has often been considered the prime factor leading to changes in the infant's gut microbiome from a low- diverse gut microbiome dominated by *Bifidobacterium*, especially in breastfed infants, to a more diverse, stable microbiome. One recent study in 903 children from 3 to 46 months of age has shown that cessation of breastfeeding is what leads to faster maturation of the gut microbiome and not the introduction of solid and liquid foods.[22] After 2–3 years the infant's microbiome reaches a more stable, adult-like microbiome.

Bacteria found in breast milk include beneficial microbes like *Lactobacillus* and *Bifidobacterium*, but also skin bacteria, and surprisingly, bacteria that are normally found in the gut. The source of these microbes is not yet clearly understood, but different theories have been proposed.[23] It is possible that the infant's mouth and regurgitation reflexes might provide microbes that colonize the mother's milk ducts, and account for some of the bacteria present in breast milk. However, colostrum—the first milk produced by lactating mothers—has also been shown to contain bacteria, and indeed, so has breast tissue. It has been proposed that bacteria can travel from the mother's gastrointestinal tract to the breast via the lymph node system. The complete picture may involve a combination of both these events, but this is an area that requires further research, as well as understanding how these bacteria are present inside the body but do not stimulate an immune reaction.

Infants born in low-income settings may be exposed to additional unfavorable factors such as undernutrition, exposure to contaminated water, poor sanitation, and poor hygiene that can perturb their growth and the development of their gut microbiome.

While there are many factors influencing the early development of the gut microbiome, time of birth is also an intriguing factor.

Preterm Infants are at Risk of Necrotizing Enterocolitis and Sepsis Due to Premature Microbiome Development

Preterm infants are infants born before 37 weeks of pregnancy. These infants are affected by complications associated with prematurity such as impaired development of gut microbiome, gastrointestinal tract and immune system, and other complications associated with growth such as weight gain and delayed organ development. Infants born prematurely before 32 weeks of pregnancy and especially those with very low weight are transferred to a special ward within the hospital called the neonatal intensive care unit and put on a special feeding routine to help them gain weight.[24] In some hospitals, preterm infants are given antibiotics as prevention to keep the risk of infection as low as possible because they are at high risk of developing life-threatening conditions such as necrotizing enterocolitis and sepsis.[25] Depending from hospital to hospital, the feeding routine is different, but in most cases is a combination of breastmilk, sometimes pasteurized, with formula milk and occasionally supplemented with probiotics.

As opposed to term infants, the gut microbiota of preterm infants is characterized by delayed colonization, limited microbial diversity, and increased abundance of pathogenic and facultative anaerobic bacteria such as *Enterobacter*, *Enterococcus*, *Escherichia*, and *Klebsiella*. Similar to term infants, the development of the gut microbiome in preterm infants is also influenced by the mode of delivery, antibiotic use, and feeding type.

Necrotizing enterocolitis is a serious gastrointestinal problem that affects 5–10 percent of premature infants born before 32 weeks of pregnancy. The condition happens when the tissue in the small or large intestine is injured or inflamed leading to intestinal damage and even death of the intestinal tissue. In some cases, a hole may form in the intestine and the bacteria can leak through and reach the abdomen or enter the bloodstream causing infections, sometimes leading to sepsis. Sepsis is the body's overreaction and a toxic response to an infection. This overreaction response of the immune system can lead to more tissue damage, organ failure, and even death.

Necrotizing enterocolitis usually develops within 3–6 weeks after birth of preterm infant. The specific cause of this condition is not properly understood, but the increased abundance of pathogenic bacteria in the intestine, immaturity of the intestine, immune system and gut microbiome, and prolonged use of antibiotics are some of the factors associated with the development of necrotizing enterocolitis. It is not entirely understood how exactly the microbiome is involved in the development of this condition. However scientific studies have shown that low microbial diversity together with the predominance of a single bacterial genus belonging to the Proteobacteria phylum could be leading to it. The abundance of these single Proteobacteria genus may trigger an overreaction of the immune system in the gut, which leads to intestinal damage and the onset of necrotizing enterocolitis.[26] In one study, scientists observed that preterm infants born before 32 weeks of pregnancy who have a higher gut microbiome diversity and abundance of *Bifidobacterium* in their gut are at lower risk of developing necrotizing enterocolitis.[27]

Prevention and Future Directions

Necrotizing enterocolitis and sepsis cause the highest number of deaths in preterm infants and lead to severe problems in the survivors, and therefore there is an increased need for preventive measures that can reduce the risk of preterm infants developing these diseases.

An abnormal gut microbiome characterized by low diversity and decreased abundance of beneficial bacteria can predispose preterm infants to develop these life-threatening diseases. Therefore, modulating the preterm infant's gut microbiome through breastfeeding or administration of breastmilk, including additional supplementation with probiotics may reduce the disease risk in preterm infants.

As mentioned in this section, breastmilk is composed of many nutrients for both the infant and its microbiome and contains additionally antimicrobial and other molecules that can modulate the immune system, thus being the natural option to modulate the gut microbiome and help infants grow.[28] One study involving more than 1,200 preterm infants showed that infants fed breastmilk either alone or in combinations with formula had a decreased risk of developing necrotizing enterocolitis.[29] Furthermore, a meta-analysis study that compared the results from 63 clinical trials involving more than 15,000 infants showed that probiotic supplementation with combinations of one or more *Lactobacillus* strains or one or more *Bifidobacterium* strains was better than other probiotic combinations in preventing the development of infections and especially of necrotizing enterocolitis in preterm infants at risk.[30]

Modulation of the gut microbiome is one way how the health of preterm infants can be maintained, but further study is required to understand the causes that lead to preterm birth and how it can be prevented. Developing prediction models that help detect the possibility of preterm birth early on would provide physicians the right tools to identify the risks and intervene to prolong gestation in utero and improve the health of infants after birth. A company named Ultrasound AI has developed the software Preterm AI, which can compare ultrasound images to detect changes indicating an increased risk of preterm birth. This software has been applied to real-world data in a clinical context where it was able to predict with an accuracy of over 90% preterm births and term births based on ultrasound scans performed during pregnancy.[31]

CHAPTER 11

ENHANCED QUALITY OF LIFE?

Microbiome and General Well-Being (Mood, Sleep, Weight Management)

WE live with our microcosmos, trillions of microbes in and on us, but also with our macrocosms: on our planet which rotates in space, around itself, and the sun. All living beings on planet Earth evolved to live in harmony with changes of day and night, of tide, of seasons, and of years. There is a clock in every living cell, also known as a "circadian clock"—for Latin words "circa" (around) and "diem" (a day).

We all know how wonderful we feel after a night of good sleep whereas a night of bad sleep can ruin the next day, or sometimes several days. Those who have taken long flights to the east or west are well familiar with "jet lags".

The main hormone in our body responsible for good sleep is melatonin. It is produced in our brain by our pituitary gland. This hormone is made by the transformation of another chemical (also a hormone and neurotransmitter)—serotonin. Serotonin is responsible for various processes in our body; from the proper functioning of our blood system, liver, gut movements, wound healing, sexual functions, pain sensation, and general mood and behavior. When the serotonin levels in the blood are normal, we feel calm, happy, focused, and stable. If it is too low, we tend to suffer from bad sleep, anxiety, and depression. Too high serotonin is also not good as it leads to overexcitation, diarrhea, fever, and even seizures. Many of the current drugs, both therapeutical and recreational, exert their effect by targeting serotonin metabolism. More than 90 percent of serotonin in our body is produced by special kinds of cells in the gut wall, the so-called enterochromaffin cells (EC), and only less than 10 percent in neurons and other cells.[1]

Germ-free, or GF mice (see Chapter 3) have serotonin levels far below normal. Practical experiments conducted by scientists display that by directly communicating to the cells in the gut (EC), introducing gut bacteria into GF mice elevates serotonin levels. Furthermore, they found that specific bacteria-produced metabolites are responsible for this effect.[2]

An increasing number of publications confirm links between sleep quality, sleep disorders and the gut microbiome diversity, and more precisely, specific types of microbes and/or metabolites they produce. Some sleep disorders, such as sleep breath disorder (SBD) or obstructive sleep apnea (OSA) affect various organ systems and can be serious, even life-threatening.[3]

There is a sophisticated interplay between our gut microbiome and the circadian rhythm. For example, depending on the time of the day, there are changes in levels of certain bacteria in our gut. Microbes adjust their metabolic activities to our phases of activity or rest.[4]

We have learned previously that the so-called microbiome-gut-brain-axis is bidirectional. Practically, it means that a disturbance of sleep or circadian rhythm can affect the gut microbiome and vice versa.

Microbiome interventions for the improvement of sleep quality and/or treatment of sleep disorders are an appealing alternative to the current pharmacological approaches. They could include the application of special probiotic strains, known to affect psychophysical well-being and behavior, also popularly called "psychobiotics". Another alternative is the use of microbial metabolites. However, more knowledge regarding microbial marker species and metabolites is required to address this question in larger human studies. In the experiments on animals, it has been shown that feeding times and type of diet have a major influence on circadian rhythms. Any eventual microbiome intervention, with probiotics or similar, needs to take this into account.

The Connections Between Weight and the Gut Microbiome

Similarly, gut microbes and their metabolites also play an important role in energy metabolism and the regulation of our weight, appetite, and energy harvest. Let's discuss some facts known about the connections between diet, microbiome, and metabolic health.

1.   Interpreting the Firmicutes/Bacteroidetes ratio

Several studies comparing the microbiota of obese and lean people conclude that obese people are characterized by lower microbial diversity in the gut and a **higher Firmicutes/Bacteroidetes ratio**. Firmicutes are a broad group of bacteria including important butyrate producers, as well as *Lactobacillus* and Clostridia. Importantly, Firmicutes are able to harvest more energy from food and deliver the host more energy following their own degradation of the nutrients in the gut.[5] When much above 40 percent, Firmicutes become a marker of a predisposition to obesity. Bacteroidetes are a less diverse group abundant in the Western lifestyle and vegetarians and known to produce propionate.

Actually, 90–95 percent of all known bacteria in our gut belong to one of these two bacterial types (phyla).

Alanna Collen in her book *10% Human*[6] explained the difference in these gut microbes amounts to roughly 2 percent more calories absorbed per day (40 to 50 calories for an average diet). A quick calculation means a lean person would put on 1 kg every five months. At this rhythm, a healthy weight becomes overweight in five years and obese in ten, just because of the microbiota markup.

But this could even be underestimated. A magnificent study published in 2011[7] looking precisely at the calories in and out estimates that for an increase of just 20 percent in Firmicutes, the additional energy harvest amounts to 150 calories per day!

It is possible to use the diet to affect this Firmicutes/Bacteroidetes ratio.[8]

How does the Diet Regulate Firmicutes/Bacteroidetes?

One hypothesis is that as Firmicutes are more efficient in harvesting energy from food than Bacteroidetes, when carbohydrates are in abundance, they will produce short-chain fatty acids in excess, increasing local acidity. Firmicutes, which are more tolerant to acidity, will thrive, while Bacteroidetes, which are more sensitive, will sense pH reduction and will stop feeding to preserve themselves. As a consequence, more calories from food will be absorbed.[9]

So, the more we eat, the more we favor Firmicutes to the detriment of Bacteroidetes, and the more they will harvest energy from our food intake. Vicious cycle, isn't it?

Additionally, as we mentioned in the previous chapter, chemicals produced by the gut microbes indirectly (e.g. by peptides secreted by the gut wall) regulate our blood sugar level and our feeling of appetite or satiety.

2. TMAO: for better or for worse

A high-fat diet rich in animal products such as meat, cheese, and eggs brings in choline, phosphatidylcholine, and L-carnitine. Although not problematic per se, when these compounds go through the process of digestion and are processed by the gut microbiota, they transform into trimethylamine (TMA). In turn, trimethylamine in the liver is oxidized into trimethylamine-N-oxide (TMAO), a compound known for its toxicity and proatherogenic property: it increases the risks of arterial hardening, clogs, and cardiovascular disease.[10]

Studies have determined the microbial culprits responsible for these metabolic conversions[11] and even proposed probiotics to reduce these bacteria and their pathways.

If the bacteria thriving on these foods no longer receive substantial amounts of nutrients, their abundance will naturally decrease, and they will be less numerous to transform your once-in-a-week rib-eye into stiff arteries.

Reducing red meat, liver, poultry, fish, milk, and cheese in favor of more plant-based foods brings additional benefits to your microbiota and cardiovascular health as well as the planet.[12]

3.   ClpB: a microbial metabolite slips into hormonal regulation of appetite

New studies conducted with state-of-the-art sequencing methods identify microbial markers in fecal samples down to the genes expressed and metabolites produced by bacteria. Such a study recently found a negative correlation between the abundance of bacterial metabolite Caseinolytic peptidase B (ClpB) and Body-Mass-Index (BMI).[13] In other words, the leaner the participants, the more ClpB was present in their feces.

ClpB has been described as a conformational antigen mimetic of alpha-MSH, one of the key hormones regulating **appetite**.[14] As ClpB presents a homology of sequence and structure to alpha-MSH, it activates the hormone's **receptor**,[15] which up-signals feeling of fullness.

The cause-to-effect relationship has been demonstrated in mice **studies**[16] and in overweight **adults**[17] to confirm that the intake of a specific probiotic able to produce ClpB helps reduce appetite and food intake, and supports weight loss.

Conclusion

Diet impacts the microbiota, which in turn impacts health status, metabolism, and weight. There's a good chance that the diet acts as a double sword: eat well, and the microbiota will exert protective effects. But if you eat too much food, too much fat, or too many animal products, you probably select a microbiota with deleterious effects which will further impact your weight gain, atherosclerosis, and even possibly increase your appetite.

This is empowering and gives room for optimism because studies show a change in diet has an almost immediate impact on the microbiota[18] (although it can take about a year to normalize levels of Firmicutes/Bacteroidetes.[19] Basically, if you go on a diet, you don't do it only for yourself, but also for the balance of your microbial community, and once the community turns friendly, it will make your efforts easier and more fruitful.

Beyond how the diet impacts the microbiome and weight management efforts, many probiotics were developed to support weight loss, cholesterol homeostasis, and even improve blood glucose metabolism in type 2 diabetes—with more or less clinical efficacy and relevance. A new generation of probiotic strains is also being evaluated for future therapeutic potential,[20] including under a drug status, so the world could change towards much more microbiome and probiotic attention in the medical management of weight and metabolic health. More about probiotics we will discuss in Chapter 13.

What Happens When We Exercise!

> *"Wer rastet der rostet"* ("Who rests rusts")
>
> —old German proverb

With the invention of cars and, especially computers, *Homo sapiens* have become more sedentary, especially since a few decades. Our ancestors had to walk tens of kilometers a day to obtain food and do other daily activities. And this current lifestyle is driving many businesses such as physiotherapy, numerous fitness programs, and apps for smartphones.

We know that exercise improves the function of the most important muscle in our body: our heart. Without oxygen, the human brain can function only for a few minutes. Better heart function means more oxygen for our brain and we feel and think better. On top of it, physical activity improves our blood circulation, immune system, nervous system, and others. In other words, it improves our general health and well-being.

As we learn more and more about the mutual interplay between food, microbiomes, and different parts of our body, there is a growing interest in finding links between our physical activity, microbiomes, and nutrition. Questions are, if, and how exactly physical activity influences our microbiomes, and by which mechanism? And vice versa, how the changes in our microbiomes, for example by certain diets or food supplements, can influence our fitness level? The latter is particularly of interest if a higher level of physical activity is required, such as in competitive sports.

Multiple studies compared, for example, gut microbiome changes between sedentary lifestyle, light, moderate, or intense physical activity. A common conclusion is that the overall abundance and diversity of bacteria in the gut increases with an increased level of exercise.[21] Certainly, there are some limitations. Extremely strenuous and prolonged physical efforts, such as in performance athletes, have shown negative effects of increasing gut permeability and leakage of bacteria through the gut-blood barrier, increasing inflammation.[22]

Comparative studies of gut microbiomes between different types of physical activities and sports range from marathon runners (half- or full-marathon), Olympic athletes, cyclists, swimmers, professional rugby players, and bodybuilders, to martial art fighters. In some cases, an increase of specific bacteria has been observed (such as *Prevotella* or *Akkermansia* in cyclists, or *Veillonella* in marathon runners). However, in many others (such as between swimmers or different Olympic disciplines), there was no change in bacterial diversity, whereas in bodybuilders it was difficult to distinguish between the effects of exercise and special nutrition.[23]

Similar to the other microbiome studies, to be able to understand the complex interplay between our microbiomes and exercise, we need to understand the role of individual microbes in the communities and how they influence fitness. From a relatively limited number of studies, it seems that the active lifestyle increases the abundance of exactly those bacterial gut species also known as probiotics (e.g. *Bifidobacteria, Lactobacillus*), as well as of short-chain fatty acid-producing bacterial species. However, it is often a challenging task to link an increase or decrease of a particular bacterial type (taxa) or a metabolite to a given metabolic pathway. For example, *Veillonella* was increased in marathon runners after the race and additional experiments confirmed that it also increased physical endurance in mice. One possibility is that the observed effect is due to an alternative metabolism of lactic acid by this bacterium, which is produced in excess by our muscles after a strenuous physical activity such as a marathon run. Future human and animal studies on the functional roles of various members of the gut microbiome should shed more light on such questions.

In the previous section we mentioned the complexity of relations between gut microbiome and nutrition, as well as the booming branch of gut microbiome-based personalized nutritional advice. Professional sports and the activities requiring advanced physical performances add another layer of complexity to it. Personalized nutrition for elite athletes, combined with special probiotic strains, should answer the following questions: how to improve endurance and absorption of key nutrients?[24] How to mitigate inflammation and a loss of immunity under hard environmental conditions? How to achieve faster recovery after intense physical activity or an injury? How to improve sleep and mood? Several startup companies, such as Boston-based Fitbiomics, or Berlin-based Prevess, already address these questions.

Microbes Can Help Prolong Our Lives?

Since ancient times, people have tried to prolong human life, or find a mythical "elixir of youth". More than a hundred years ago (1907), in his book *Prolongation of Life: Optimistic Studies*, the father of immunology Elie Metchnikoff discussed the reasons for extremely long human life. Taking historical examples of centenarians for whom drinking excess alcohol or smoking most of their lives was quite normal, his conclusion was that no single factor can be used as a prognostic marker for longevity. On the other hand, similar to Hippocrates, (the "father" of modern medicine who claimed more than 2,000 years ago that "all disease start in the gut"), Metchnikoff also hypothesized that due to the relatively large size of the colon in humans, there is more space for the microbe-assisted processes of food decomposition and fermentation, producing substances which can be harmful to the body. His advice, which he actually followed himself throughout his later life, was daily consumption of sour milk and yogurt made by fermentation with cultures of lactic acid bacteria (e.g. *Lactobacillus bulgaricus*) which he thought counteracted the negative effects of food decay in the gut, therefore prolonging life. As support for his idea, he found an above-average number of centenarians in Eastern Europe at that time.[25] Although Metchnikoff didn't reach the age of 100 (he died at age 71 from heart failure), nowadays we know that numerous strains of lactic acid bacteria actually do have beneficial health effects, a topic which we will discuss later in the chapter about probiotics.

But What Does Aging Actually Mean?

In general, scientists agree that each person has two different kinds of ages: the chronological age (calculated from our birthdate) and the biological one. There are various methods to estimate the biological age, taking into account multiple parameters, such as the status of blood vessels, hormones, and metabolites in the body, the number of mutations in body cells or length of specific DNA repeats on human chromosomes, called telomeres (which become shorter by aging) and many others. Since recently, the gut microbiome is also considered a good aging marker and a target for anti-aging interventions.[26] It is reasoned by a general decline in gut microbiome diversity with aging and, as we previously discussed, connections between the microbiome and immune system. Aging of the immune system (immunosenescence) combined with the lower microbiome diversity, leads to long-term, low-grade inflammation, potentially contributing to many health conditions in the body, a process called "Inflammaging". Second, centenarians seem to have distinctive microbiome profiles, different from young people but also from, for example, a 70-year-old. A recent study in Japan, known for its above-average population of centenarians, found increased levels of a unique chemical (a secondary bile acid) produced by gut microbes.[27] Beyond leading a generally healthy lifestyle (e.g. moderate physical activity, reduction of stress, toxins, etc.), scientists are trying to create microbiome-based anti-aging treatments based on a special diet, use of specific bacterial strains, or their mixtures (probiotics or microbial stool transplants, see later).[28] A company called Deep Longevity has been recently granted a patent to determine a person's age based on the gut microbiome.[29]

Mitochondria as Ancient Microbial "Powerplants"

An interesting potential mechanism of improving our body's performance is actually via small energy "powerplants" in each of our cells, called **mitochondria**. As per now generally accepted theory, mitochondria themselves were once ancient bacteria trapped by cells of virtually all multicellular organisms, creating a symbiotic relationship.

Unlike genes that we inherit from both of our parents, we inherit mitochondria only from our mothers.

The main function of mitochondria is to produce a molecule called Adenosine Triphosphate (ATP) which is the fuel for all molecular processes in our body. ATP formation is the final stage of burning sugars in our cells and, similar to burning fuel in our cars, it needs oxygen. However, molecules known as "free radicals" or "reactive oxygen species" (ROS) are formed in this process (as well as taken into our body externally through various toxic compounds we ingest or inhale), damaging our cells and in particular, mitochondria.

Without going into details, the more ROS in our cells, the more mutations accumulate in our mitochondria, increasing the risk for various diseases and accelerating our aging.[30] Therefore, mitochondria can be used as overall body health and aging *biomarker* (explained in Chapter 13), the opportunity already commercially used by some companies. Others are promising to improve health by improving the function of mitochondria.

By influencing each cell in our body, mitochondria inevitably influence cells in our gut and therefore also our gut microbiome. On the other hand, our gut microbiome can influence the formation of ROS, therefore can indirectly influence our mitochondrial health in a positive or a negative way.[31]

Isn't it amazing that we actually stay young, fit, and healthy when our extracellular microbes communicate well with our intracellular microbes!

PART IV

HUMAN MICROBIOMES IN EVERYDAY LIFE (APPLICATIONS)

CHAPTER 12

SCALING THE MICROBIOME ENTREPRENEURSHIP

SUPPORTED by landmark research projects and findings, surging venture investments, and an uptick in pharma and biotech's microbiome therapeutic pipeline, the microbiome market is growing at a rapid pace. Let's peel back the layers and look at the macro indicators.

Publication of scientific papers focused on microbiome research has been surging with over 75,000 publications and steady growth of more than 20 percent in the past three years (as shown in figure 1 below). It is believed that 90 percent of diseases can be linked in some way back to the gut and the health of the microbiome and research has shown that the microbiome is more medically accessible and manipulable than the human genome.[1] This has resulted in a dramatic rise in microbiome research which in turn is driven by advances in next-generation sequencing (NGS), bioinformatics, synthetic biology, metabolomics, and significant reductions in the cost of sequencing.

Microbiome research grants continue to increase with $1 billion being awarded to research in the area (as seen in figure 2). Several pioneering studies from 2006 including landmark projects such as the Human Microbiome Project and EU MetaHit (METAgenomics of the Human Intestinal Tract) project, laid the foundation for this field, showing an upward trend till 2019. For the first time, there was a

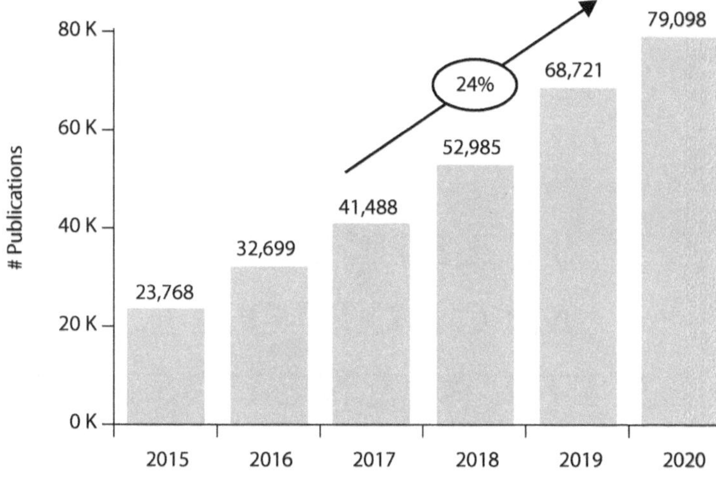

Figure 12.1   Microbiome Publications Trend

Source: Arogyam Analytics of the Microbiome Whitepaper

marked dip in funding amount in 2020. Funding dropped from ~$1.9 billion in 2019 to ~$1.1 billion in 2020, impacted by COVID. One could expect 2022to catch up and reflect the five years upward trend from 2015–2019.

The number of ongoing clinical trials with a focus on the microbiome has risen substantially from 2015 to 2019 to ~190 trials while 2020 was impacted by COVID (as seen in figure 3). A majority of these can be expected to be reinitiated.

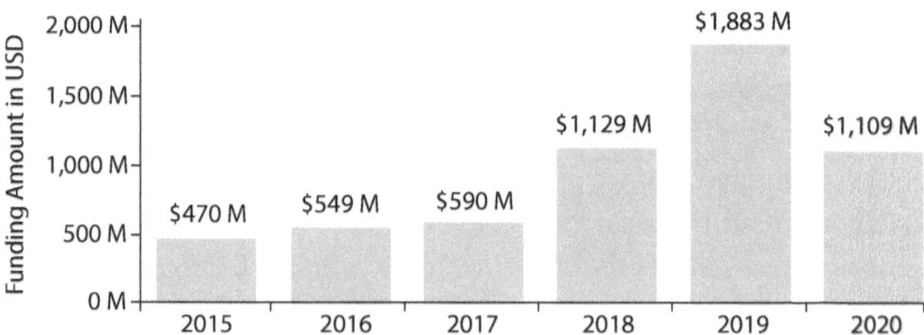

Figure 12.2   Microbiome Grants Trend

Source: Arogyam Analytics of the Microbiome Whitepaper

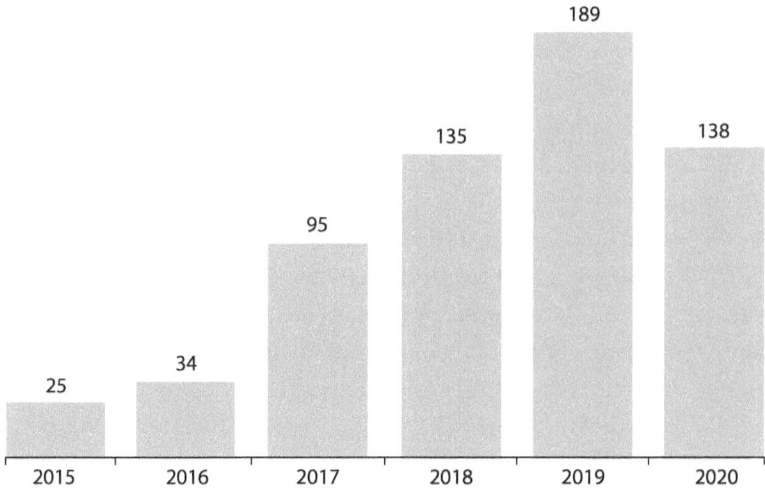

Figure 12.3   Number of Ongoing Clinical Trials Examining the Microbiome

Source: Arogyam Analytics of the Microbiome Whitepaper

Positive gains in later-stage clinical trials have spurred the industry. Success in gastrointestinal (GI) diseases from Seres, Finch, Rebiotix, and Vedanta is noteworthy. Cancer has been another area that has seen increased clinical trial activity in utilizing microbiome research for cancer drugs. The microbiome is believed to be a key enabler of response to immunotherapies, a Nobel prize-winning cancer treatment. This has led to several collaborations between large pharmaceutical companies and microbiome companies building microbiome therapies. Some noteworthy examples would be Merck's collaboration with 4D pharma to test their microbiome intervention with Merck's blockbuster immunotherapy drug, Keytruda, Bristol-Myers Squibb's immunotherapy collaboration with Enterome, and Rebiotix's acquisition by Ferring Pharmaceuticals in 2018.

These breakthroughs are likely to pave the way for other indications such as autoimmune diseases, neuropsychiatric and neuro-degenerative diseases, infectious and skin diseases. Personalized microbiome-directed therapies are likely to be the next frontier.

However, uncertainties from regulatory bodies regarding classification and frameworks for microbiome therapeutics are likely to remain a barrier.

Exponential growth in venture investment into startup companies in the microbiome market has been observed. Investors are betting big on microbiome companies, 2020 saw close to $2 billion being raised by startup companies (see figure 4).

The proliferation of startups in therapeutics and food has led the way. Therapeutics companies, buoyed by success in clinical trials have consistently received funding. Besides companies in the GI area in the therapeutics category, companies focused on oncology, neurology, metabolic and skin diseases have also received investors' attention. For instance, Kallyope focused on gut–brain axis has raised $480 million to date while skin microbiome company Azitra, has received $40 million in funding to date. Enterome, which employs "-omics" platforms to generate precision drugs, has raised $130 million. Building a consistent drug product from the various therapeutic approaches requires time and investment. This is where a reliable contract development and manufacturing company (CDMO) with the ability to manufacture microbiome therapeutics will be important. CDMOs like Arranta Bio are garnering attention as well, raising $85 million. Leading investors on the therapeutic front are Seventure Partners, JLabs, Khosla Ventures, and Leaps (Bayer).

Diagnostics companies utilizing NGS and advanced machine learning such as Karius have raised a substantial $245 million to date

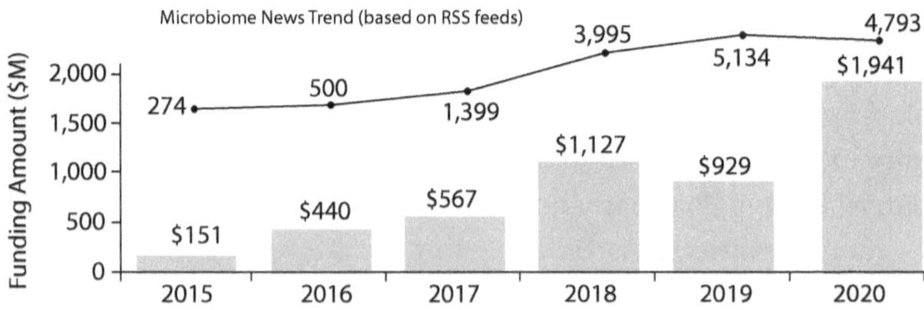

Figure 12.4   Investments in Microbiome Companies Over Time ($M)

Source: Arogyam Analytics of the Microbiome Whitepaper

for hypothesis-free clinical infectious testing. The explosion of public awareness of consumer DNA testing such as ancestry and probiotic supplements has led to the rise of a plethora of consumer gut microbiome testing companies to guide precision nutrition such as Viome, Thryve, Flore (Sun Genomics), and DayTwo. Viome leads the pack having raised $105 million to date. Vivante Health is an interesting digital health company leveraging microbiome research in its digital gut health program and has raised about $40 million to date.

The functional foods category such as probiotics, prebiotics, and others to establish a healthy microbiome have received ample funding. Perfect Day, a producer of animal-free milk substitutes and proteins that are nutritionally identical to cow's milk, leads the pack with an impressive haul of ~$365 million to date.

Consumer-facing skincare has seen increasing attention being paid to the microbiome on the skin. AOBiome's consumer division, Mother Dirt saw a meteoric rise of their AO+ Mist containing the live culture of ammonia-oxidizing bacteria which harmonizes the ecosystem on one's skin. AOBiome has raised $40 million to date.

In conclusion, there is continued progress and explosive potential from growing research, awareness, and a well-funded ecosystem of companies. All signs point to the microbiome market evolving into a powerhouse of interventions for human health.

Microbiome Therapeutics Companies—Trying to Fuel New Alternatives to Treat Disease

The various start-ups in the microbiome therapeutics space are trying to harness the power of the microbiome in treating various diseases. New research in the field of the microbiome suggests that microbiota are intricately related to the health and wellness of an individual. And this is the premise that many microbiome therapeutics companies are trying to base their solutions on. Microbiome therapeutics deal with various means by which the microbiota can be modulated or with finding molecules produced by microbiota that can be used for therapeutic purposes.

> **Various means for modulating microbiota**
>
> A) Live therapeutics: Inclusion of specially derived microbes with known effects on a particular disease or complementing other kinds of therapy (e.g. cancer immunotherapy).
> B) Small molecules: Small molecules affecting the microbiota or their interaction with the host.[2]
> C) Peptides: These are short chain of amino acids that may modulate the microbiota.[3]
> D) Genetically modified microbes: these microbes are genetically modified to carry certain genes that can be directed against certain diseases.
> E) Bacteriophages: viruses that specifically infect or kill a certain type of bacteria.

Most of the companies are in the research and development phase or early phase clinical trial stage and several have advanced into the late-stage human clinical trial. The appended box will provide the reader with some idea about the companies that are fueling the microbiome therapeutics domain. This isn't an exhaustive list.

Companies Active in Microbiome Therapeutics

> Company Name – Seres Therapeutics
>
> Country – USA
>
> Pipeline – Based on the approach of using multifunctional consortia of bacteria
>
> SER-109 – *Clostridium difficile* infection
>
> SER -301 – Ulcerative colitis

Company Name – Rebiotix, a Ferring Pharmaceutical company

Country – USA

Pipeline – Based on the approach of using multifunctional consortia of bacteria

RBX2660 – *Clostridium difficile* infection

Company Name – Finch Therapeutics

Country – USA

Pipeline – Based on the approach of using multifunctional consortia of bacteria

CP101 – *Clostridium difficile* infection

FIN525 – Crohn's disease

TAK-524 – Ulcerative colitis

FIN-211 – Autism spectrum disorder

Company Name – Enterome Biosciences

Country – France

Pipeline – Peptide therapeutics based on the gut microbiota

TAK-018 – Crohn's disease

E02401 – Cancer (glioblastoma and adrenal tumors)

Company Name – Vedanta Biosciences

Country – USA

Pipeline – Based on the approach of using multifunctional consortia of bacteria

VE303 – *C.difficile* infection

VE202 – Inflammatory bowel disease

VE800 – Solid tumors

Company Name – Maat Pharma

Country – France

Pipeline – Oncology focused; based on the approach of using multi-functional consortia of bacteria

MaaT013 – Graft versus host disease, melanoma

Company Name – Axial Therapeutics

Country – US

Pipeline – Microbiome gut–brain axis focused; based on gut microbiome targeted small molecule therapeutics

AB 2004 – Autism associated irritability

AB 5006 – Parkinson's disease

Company Name – BiomX

Country – Israel

Pipeline – Based on natural and engineered phage therapy

BX 004 – Cystic fibrosis

BX 005 – Atopic dermatitis

BX 003 – Inflammatory bowel disease

Company Name – Ysopia Bioscience

Country – France

Pipeline – Based on single strain live biotherapeutics

Yso 1 – Obesity and metabolic disorders

Yso 2 – Crohn's disease

BX 003 – Inflammatory bowel disease

Company Name – KoBioLabs

Country – South Korea

Pipeline – Based on live biotherapeutics

KBL 697 – Inflammatory bowel disease

KBL 693 – Atopic dermatitis

Company Name – Kaleido Bioscience

Country – USA

Pipeline – Chemistry-driven synthetic molecules targeting the micro-biome

KB295 – Ulcerative colitis

KB109 – Chronic obstructive pulmonary disease

Company Name – Evelo

Country – USA

Pipeline – Single strain of non-live microbes or their vesicles targeting the small intestine axis with a focus on inflammatory diseases

EDP1815 – Psoriasis, atopic dermatitis

The above list was a snapshot of the various companies active in the domain of microbiome therapeutics. There are a few companies that are trying to base their products on "fecal microbiota transplantation" or FMT, the process of transferring the microbes from a healthy donor to a patient. One of the companies in this domain is EnteroBiotix, UK.

CHAPTER 13

PREBIOTICS, PROBIOTICS, POSTBIOTICS, AND SYNBIOTICS

THE concept that certain nutrients can selectively modify the gut microbiota exists for a long time. The first reports showing the bifidogenic effect of insulin and other oligosaccharides were first published in the 1980s. But, scientists already described in the 1950s, the existence of the "bifidus factor" in human milk which enriches the abundance of *Bifidobacterium* species in infants.[1]

Even before the scientific world introduced the word probiotic, it was in vogue for several decades in the form of fermented food and products such as kefir, kombucha, sauerkraut, bread, wine, beer, and cheese. These products had been used by households very frequently. In Latin 'pro' stands for 'for' and 'biotic' stands for 'life'. In short, probiotic can be considered for life.

In Chapter 6 we introduced the terms eubiosis and dysbiosis as two important states of the microbiome that are strongly associated with various health-related outcomes. We have highlighted that external factors such as a diet rich in ultra-processed foods, fats, sugars and additives, smoking, alcohol, stress, antibiotics, and medication can cause disbalance in the gut microbiota and lead to digestive problems such as diarrhea, constipation, bloating, and abdominal pain. It can also result in more serious diseases like obesity, diabetes, and other gastrointestinal disorders.[2] One way to support the restoration of healthy balance and especially the recovery of the eubiosis state is through the administration of biotics.[3] In case of severe symptoms, medication can be recommended, although most medications treat the symptoms but not the cause. Another way to restore microbial composition is through nourishing the microbiome with foods rich in prebiotics and other fibers and maintaining a healthy lifestyle.

In this chapter, we will be discussing probiotics, prebiotics, synbiotics, and postbiotics.

Probiotics are defined by the International Scientific Association for Probiotics and Prebiotics (ISAPP) as "live microorganisms that, when administered in adequate amounts, confer a health benefit on the host."[4] The probiotics are known by genus, species, and strain; for example, for *Lactobacillus acidophilus* LA-5, *Lactobacillus* is the name of the genus, *acidophilus* is the name of the species, LA-5 indicates the strain. The strain designation is important for each probiotic because different strains of the same species confer different health benefits. Microorganisms qualify as probiotics if they are well characterized by genomic sequencing and strain level identification, are safe to use, have been shown to confer at least one health benefit in one human study, or belong to species that are well recognized for their beneficial effects. Probiotics have been shown to have many different beneficial effects, but do note that not all probiotic strains will have the same beneficial effects. To name a few of their positive effects, probiotics can help in reducing the incidence and duration of antibiotic-associated diarrhea, in managing digestive discomfort, in reducing symptoms of lactose maldigestion, and can decrease the risk or duration of upper respiratory tract infections (such as a common cold) or gut infections.

Probiotics can be included in different products, such as food, capsules, tablets, shots, and even gummy bears to support a healthy gut and often to address other health needs, such as reducing stress and helping with weight management, for women's health and many more. In supermarkets or even online shops, you might come across different foods that contain probiotics such as chocolate, cereals, sports drinks, baby food, yogurt, ice cream, and many more. Depending on the country where you are located, the term "probiotic" may even be present on the product label. In Europe, the European Commission considers the term "probiotic" as a health claim, and although there have been many applications for health claims for probiotics, until now, no health claims have been approved for probiotics. There are a few countries that allow the use of the "probiotic" term on product labels such as Italy, Spain, and Denmark.[5]

Many of the probiotic strains available on the market belong to the *Bifidobacterium* and *Lactobacillus* genera, but there are a few other strains belonging to genera such as *Bacillus, Streptococcus, Enterococcus, Pediococcus, Escherichia coli, Lactococcus, Pediococcus, Leuconostoc,* and even some yeasts, like *Saccharomyces,* that have been shown to provide health benefits when consumed in adequate amounts.[6]

Both *Bifidobacterium* and *Lactobacillus* species are normal inhabitants of the healthy human microbiome and are considered beneficial microorganisms.

Bifidobacterium genus is associated with the diversity and robustness of the gut microbiota, and is one of the dominant groups of microorganisms in the gut, together with other genera such as *Ruminococcus, Blautia, Roseburia, Anaerostipes, Lachnospiraceae, Faecalibacterium, Bacteroides,* etc.[7] *Bifidobacterium* species are among the first microbes to colonize the human gastrointestinal tract and are highly abundant in breast-fed infants and play an important role as the first microbes to colonize the gut being involved in training the immune system, preventing pathogens from invading and breaking the mother's milk into beneficial substances for the infant's health.[8] In adults, *Bifidobacterium* accounts for up to 5 percent of the total microorganisms present in the gut, and their presence is associated with health benefits including the production of metabolites such as short-chain fatty acids (SCFAs) and vitamins, prevention of gut disorders, and immune system development.[9]

Lactobacillus are members of the Lactic Acid Bacteria (LAB), a group characterized by the formation of lactic acid as the only or main end product of their carbohydrate metabolism. Lactobacillus are only a minor member of the gut microbiome with a prevalence of 0.01 percent,[10] but they are highly abundant in other body sites, such as the small intestine, vagina, and oral cavity.[11] *Lactobacillus* species present in the gastrointestinal tract are known to have many beneficial effects on the host. These effects are linked to their capabilities of producing several important substances, including lactate (or lactic acid), SCFAs, and other antimicrobial substances which keep the pathogenic bacteria from disrupting the gut ecosystem.[12] In the small intestine, *Lactobacillus* species are producing vitamin B12, which is an essential vitamin for the human body. They also play an important role in maintaining healthy gut mucosa.[13] *Lactobacillus* species are well known for their use in fermentation processes and are often used in producing dairy products, fermented foods, sourdough, etc.

Similar to *Bifidobacterium* and *Lactobacillus* strains, *Bacillus* strains can provide different health benefits depending on the strains used in the products. The *Bacillus* strains are used in their spore form when included in products or foods, which is different from how *Bifidobacterium* and *Lactobacillus* strains are used.[14] Strains of *Lactobacillus* and *Bifidobacterium* are added to products in their living, vegetative state, meaning they are in an active form and are quite sensitive to high heat, oxygen, and even different pH conditions. Thus, limiting their application in different foods and products, while the *Bacillus* spores are quite stable to high heat treatments and different variations in pH making them suitable to be used in various foods and products. Spores are like plant seeds, they are in a dormant state and will only grow if the right temperature, moisture, and food sources are present. The spores are usually activated once they reach the small intestine, as the conditions are appropriate for germination.[15]

Probiotic strains rarely colonize the gastrointestinal tract. Colonization means that the probiotic strains can grow and thrive and remain in the gastrointestinal tract for extended periods. Imagine the large intestine like a jungle, there are so many microbes present in the entire intestine that for a new microbe to find a home to live in is not easy. The new microbe has to compete with other resident microbes for similar substrates to grow. Since the gut microbiome in adults is quite stable, new microbes from outside would have a slim chance of winning against the microbes that are already well adapted to this environment and have been there since childhood. That is why most probiotics are transient, they are present in the gut for as long as you take them, and once you stop taking the probiotics, after a few days they will not be present anymore in your gut. But, that does not mean that they do not have a beneficial effect. Probiotics are known to contribute to gut health and confer different health benefits to the host. They produce metabolites that can support the activity of the gut microbiota and can even have beneficial effects on the intestinal epithelium for instance maintaining the thickness of the mucus layer via regulation of specific genes. Furthermore, probiotics can help your gut microbiota to outcompete and eliminate pathogens. They can even modulate your immune system, and some can help your body by producing vitamins and digesting specific dietary compounds.

Next-Generation Probiotics

These are the traditional probiotics coming from the culture, in laboratories, and subsequently in industrial fermenters, of microorganisms often isolated from healthy people's feces or foods. However, these taxonomic groups are not preponderant in healthy colonic microbiota. In normal conditions, the colon, where most of the microorganisms you host are thriving, is deprived of oxygen. Co-evolution has thus favored microorganisms that prosper in anaerobic conditions—meaning in the total absence of oxygen. For these microbes, the strong oxidative power of oxygen is detrimental, or even lethal. The implication is profound: when researchers started culturing fecal samples in the lab, where the air is 20 percent rich in oxygen, these bacteria could not grow. And therefore, we missed the bulk of our microbiota altogether in the first generations of probiotics.

Due to advancements in sequencing technologies and anaerobic laboratory equipment, identification and culturing of these microorganisms that are more typical and abundant in healthy microbiota is doable. Based on these advancements, several industries are working on a new age of probiotics, referred to as next-generation probiotics. Several definitions have been proposed such as "well-characterized probiotic strains which could be used as delivery vehicles for a specific molecule abrogating the disease phenotype and thus promoting health."[16] These definitions highlight:

(1) A difference in the perception of the health benefit, here more oriented toward diseases, or "live microorganisms identified on the basis of comparative microbiota analyses that, when administered in adequate amounts, confer a health benefit on the host."[17]

(2) Pointing the finger at the next-generation method of identification rather than at the scope of use.

Usually, the terminology next-generation probiotics refer to new microorganisms that have no history of safe use (and thus will require a lot of studies to demonstrate their safety before they can be brought to the market) and are hard to grow industrially because of their sensibility to oxygen, which explains why it is taking time to see them coming to the shelves.

Little by little, however, they will bring a lot more possibilities to the probiotic world. The most famous and expected on the market are *Akkermansia muciniphila*, a mucus degrader participating through cross-feeding to the production of butyrate, already available in the United States and Turkey and expected in several European countries end of 2022, intended to bring health benefits in glucose metabolism and possibly, weight, and *Faecalibacterium prausnitzii*, a key butyrate producer with anti-inflammatory properties, which could make a big difference for people with inflammatory bowel syndrome or inflammatory bowel diseases such as Ulcerative Colitis or Crohn's Disease. A lot more are undergoing study, including species of the genus *Bacteroides*, *Clostridium*, *Eubacterium*, *Prevotella*, *Eggerthella*, and *Christensenella* just to name a few.[18] You should know that we are just scratching the surface and discovering new high-potential microorganisms every day, whether it is in human health or in massive research projects such as the Earth Microbiome Project,[19] off to characterize ecosystems communities across the planet, which will be an infinite source of new bugs, new functions, and new potential.

Prebiotics are defined by ISAPP as *"substrates that are selectively utilized by host microorganisms conferring a health benefit."*[20] Prebiotics are types of dietary ingredients that the human body cannot digest, meaning they serve as "food" for a selective group of beneficial microorganisms that live in the gastrointestinal tract, especially in the gut. By feeding the beneficial microbes in the gut, prebiotics modulates your gut microbiome for better health and contribute to health benefits such as improving gut transit time. It's the time taken by ingested food to travel through the human gut, improving calcium absorption, stimulating the immune system, regulating blood sugar, and reducing the lipid levels in the blood, and can even help in maintaining mental health.[21] Although most prebiotics are found in products taken orally or in food, they can also be included in products for the skin or vaginal tract.

Most known prebiotics are carbohydrate-based such as non-digestible oligosaccharides fructans, galactans, and insulin to name a few. These are the most common ones used in many supplements and are often included in functional foods. This may sound confusing, but imagine them as long, complex chains of sugars. Some prebiotics are naturally present in foods, such as fruits, vegetables, cereals, and grains, and are often referred to as dietary fibers. Dietary fibers are carbohydrate polymers, long chains of carbohydrates, that are neither degraded nor absorbed in the small intestine, but once they reach the colon they can be fermented or partially fermented by the gut microbiota into other end products such as short chain fatty acids (SCFAs). Not all dietary fibers are considered prebiotics, but a high intake of dietary fibers is linked to increased diversity in the gut microbiome and many other health benefits. According to different country regulations, an adult should consume between 25–28 grams of fiber per day. Low intake of dietary fibers has been linked to chronic diseases such as obesity, type 2 diabetes, colon cancer, and cardiovascular diseases.[22]

You can increase your intake of dietary fibers and even prebiotics by consuming certain foods and supplements. Fruits, vegetables, grains, and cereals are a great source of dietary fibers, some having more fibers than others, for example, bananas, apples, leeks, asparagus, onions, garlic, chicory root, Jerusalem artichokes, barley, whole oats, and flaxseeds.[23]

Other well-known prebiotics are the human milk oligosaccharides (HMOs) that are present in the mother's milk and are essential during the early development of infants and their gut microbiome.[24] These types of prebiotics are often included in babies' food such as formulas, to provide infants with the ingredients needed to develop a healthy gut microbiome.[25] Recent studies have shown that specific HMOs, for example, 2'FL (2-fucosyllactose), are also beneficial for adults as they are used by microbes of the *Bifidobacterium* group which are well known for their positive effect on the human body.[26]

Besides carbohydrate-based prebiotics, some polyphenols and polyunsaturated fatty acids can also be considered prebiotics, as they are selectively used by good gut microbes and provide beneficial effects on the human body. Polyphenols are a diverse group of compounds found naturally in fruits—especially berries, vegetables, cereals, tea, coffee, dark chocolate, cacao powder, and wine. From a chemistry perspective, all polyphenols have in their chemical structure phenolic rings. Many of the polyphenols are not absorbed in the small intestine and the majority of them reach the colon where they are being used by the gut microbiota as food and are often transformed into other end compounds such as SCFAs. Long-term consumption of foods rich in polyphenols can protect against certain diseases, for example, neurodegenerative diseases, gastrointestinal problems, cancer, cardiovascular disease, and type 2 diabetes. The protective effect of the polyphenols is thanks to their antioxidant and anti-inflammatory properties as well as their positive effect on the gut microbiome.[27]

Therefore, maintaining a diverse diet rich in dietary fibers and polyphenols is beneficial not only for your well-being but also for supporting a healthy and diverse microbiome.

Synbiotics are defined by ISAPP as "a mixture comprising live microorganisms and substrate(s) selectively utilized by host microorganisms that confers a health benefit on the host."[28] In simpler words, a synbiotic means combining probiotics with prebiotics in a formulation to provide health benefits for the host. There are two categories of synbiotics defined, complementary synbiotics and synergistic synbiotics. The complementary synbiotics are composed of probiotics and prebiotics that together provide one or more health benefits, but are not co-dependent, meaning the prebiotics do not have to be a substrate (food) for the co-administered probiotics. Synergistic synbiotics must contain prebiotics that are substrate and selectively used only by the co-administered probiotics.

The idea to combine probiotics and prebiotics in a synbiotic is that the two components should provide additional health benefits to the already positive effects provided by each component alone. The health benefits provided by synbiotics must be confirmed in human studies and it is not enough to just combine already well-studied probiotics and prebiotics together.

Postbiotics are defined as "a preparation of inanimate microorganisms and/or their components that confers a health benefit on the host."[29] It has long been known that microorganisms do not need to be alive to provide health benefits to the host.[30] Postbiotics result from living microorganisms that are killed through technological processes, for example, heat treatment, high pressure, pasteurization, and oxygen exposure for strict anaerobes, to name a few. Postbiotics do not need to be derived from probiotics only, meaning the microorganisms from which the postbiotics are prepared do not have to be previously studied for their beneficial effects in clinical studies. Furthermore, inactivated probiotics or probiotics that have lost their cell viability during product development processing or storage do not automatically classify as postbiotics. It is still required for the inactivated probiotics to be studied for their beneficial effects on the human body in clinical trials.

According to the definition, postbiotics must include non-living microbial biomass, either as intact microbial cells or cell components such as fragments or structures of cells. Besides the non-living microbial biomass, postbiotics can also include, although not necessary, microbial metabolites or end-products of their metabolism resulting from their growth on specific matrices or during the fermentation of specific matrices. Cell components or microbial metabolites which are isolated or purified do not classify as postbiotics. For example, before the ISAPP definition of postbiotics, isolated microbial metabolites such as butyrate or lactate were considered postbiotics, but with the new definition, these metabolites cannot be labeled as postbiotics.

For a product to be qualified as postbiotic several criteria have to be met: (i) the microorganisms included have to be well characterized using molecular techniques; (ii) the method used for inactivation has to be well described including the matrix or medium on which the microorganisms were grown; (iii) it has to be proven that the microorganisms are dead or not able to replicate; (iv) the health benefits provided by the postbiotic have to be confirmed in clinical trials; (v) the composition of the postbiotic preparation has to be described in detail and lastly, the safety of the postbiotic has to be assessed in human studies.

Postbiotics v/s Prebiotics

Similar to other biotics, postbiotics are also known to have a positive impact on health. Postbiotics exert their effect by acting on different levels for example, through direct interaction with the resident microbiota and the intestinal epithelial cells, through immunomodulatory and anti-inflammatory effects, by directly inhibiting the growth of pathogens, and by systemic signaling via the nervous system.

Compared to probiotics, postbiotics have several benefits. Postbiotics are considered safer to be given to vulnerable subjects, such as frail elderly and adults with a compromised immune system, and infants, especially preterm infants. Since the microorganisms in postbiotics are dead there is no risk of microbes being translocated from the gut to blood and causing problems, and there is no risk of acquisition or transfer of antibiotic resistance genes from postbiotics. In terms of stability, postbiotics are highly stable and are not sensitive to heat, oxygen, or pH conditions. Therefore, postbiotics can be used in different manufacturing processes and can be included in many formats and matrices such as functional foods, beverages, and supplements.[31]

Although several clinical studies are showing the health benefits of postbiotics there is still much to be discovered about the mechanisms driving their benefits and the components contributing to these benefits. One aspect is clear, postbiotics will bring great opportunities for biotic innovation and implementation in the nutritional world of functional foods and dietary supplements.

How to Select the Best Probiotics?

When selecting a probiotic supplement there are some things you should be aware of. First, more is not necessarily any better. Some products contain 10 different probiotic strains but this does not necessarily mean they will have a better effect than products that contain only one or two probiotic strains. Also, the number of living cells included in the product is important. On the product label, the name of the probiotic will appear followed by the number of live probiotics in the product, in CFU (colony-forming units). According to some country regulations, probiotic products should contain at least $1*10^9$ CFU per dose, but this number depends on the performed human studies showcasing the efficacy and safety of the specific probiotic strain. Always inform yourself about the probiotic product you wish to purchase before selecting one.

Secondly, you should avoid products that mention the CFU at the time of manufacture. Such labeling does not account for the number of live probiotics that will decline during storage, and instead opt for products that mention the CFU at the end of shelf-life.[32]

There are a lot of probiotic products on the shelves, very different from one another in terms of both quality and functionality. To choose the best for you, you should first define what you expect from your probiotic. Is it for general support for your microbiota? Or do you have more precise expectations? Would you prefer to have it from foods, or food supplements? Specific probiotics have been proven to support the immune system, reducing the incidence, prevalence, and severity of respiratory tract infections,[33] others have been studied and recommended for diarrhea,[34] constipation,[35] inflammatory bowel syndrome,[36] weight management,[37] atopic dermatitis,[38] acne,[39] asthma,[40] osteoporosis,[41] mental well-being,[42] fertility,[43] migraine,[44] mastitis during breastfeeding,[45] epilepsy,[46] etc. Of course, not a single strain can do all of this, so it's a matter of finding the right strain for you. To identify such strains, you may want to research on PubMed or Google Scholar, typing probiotics and the functionality you need. Also, not all strains will be available in all countries, and not always from the same brand, so even once you have identified the best strain or combination of strains for your expectations, you might have some more research to do to find the product delivering it.

In the United States and Canada, the Alliance for Education on Probiotics (AEProbio) has already done the work and produced a guide, mostly aimed at healthcare professionals, to better identify which strains and products have been studied in which population and application, and with which posology it should be recommended.[47]

In the shop, a probiotic label or package will already provide you with a lot of information to evaluate the product's quality. Infographics from the International Probiotics Association (IPA), ISAPP, and AEProbio are available on their websites[48] and all agree on the key criteria when you want to select a high-quality product:

- It must report the dosage (look for CFU or cells), indicate the daily serving size, and this enables you to check that this quantity corresponds to the amount proven effective in the studies.
- The product should indicate the microorganisms used, down to the strain level (i.e. *Lactobacillus acidophilus* IPA123)—otherwise, you are not able to check if there is any data at all on this strain.
- It should include the expiration date and conditions of storage to ensure that the quantity labeled is still alive until the end of shelf life.

- If the product is sold in a country where this is authorized, you could also find the recommended use or expected functionality, but it is not because it does not figure on the packaging that it has not been studied, it depends on the local regulation around health claims. In the European Union (EU). in particular, this is very limited, so much so that you will not even read the term "probiotic" in most EU countries, which is itself considered a non-authorized health claim.

Last but not least, you can also speak to your doctor about your issues and questions about probiotics, but don't expect them to know everything: it's a whole, very complex world, with an infinity of studies and functionalities with new publications every other day, and in most countries, until now, courses on nutrition and probiotics are not part at all of medical education. It is meant to change in the future, but there is always a lot of inertia before new discoveries make it to the general medical practice.

What is and is Not a Probiotic?

Although there is a consensus on the World Health Organization/ Food and Agriculture Organization/ISAPP definition of probiotics as "live microorganisms which when administered in adequate amounts confer a health benefit on the host,"[49] there is no common agreement on what qualifies as "adequate amounts" and "health benefits." Experts from across the industry and from ISAPP have elaborated precise criteria in 2020 to bring a better understanding of what the term probiotic implies, or should imply.[50] In particular:

- A probiotic must be characterized and identified down to the strain level. This means that if you read "*Lactobacillus acidophilus*" on a label, without the subsequent code that enables the identification of the individual strain, it is not sufficiently characterized. The characterization should also include whole-genome sequencing.
- A probiotic must be safe for the intended use.

- The health benefit must be shown in at least one positive human study - or the strain must belong to a species with a recognized benefit shared across the species (this is the case for *Lactobacillus bulgaricus* and *Streptococcus thermophilus*, the two species used to ferment yogurt, which are known to degrade lactose and recognized even by the European Food Safety Authority to "improve lactose digestion."[51]

If sticking to these criteria to qualify probiotics, almost no fermented foods or dietary microbes (kefir, kombucha, kimchi, sauerkraut, etc.) can be considered to contain probiotics. Some do not even contain live microorganisms (those cooked or pasteurized after the fermentation, for example). When they do, they seldom label the specific species, let alone strains, and second, their specific formulation has not been clinically studied for health benefits in humans. It does not mean that they do not bring health benefits—diets rich in fermented foods have been reported to enhance health, longevity, and quality of life[52], but that they have not demonstrated sufficiently precisely and specifically such benefits to claim to be probiotics. It is also important to note the wide intrinsic heterogeneity[53] in benefits from different strains and different fermented foods. It is about a gradient of certitude. In general, Western lifestyle and diet have impoverished the gut microbiota biodiversity, leading to poor health outcomes, and the integration of dietary microbes is reckoned to be positive in reestablishing diversity and resilience. However, the term probiotic refers to more precise and established health benefits. Yes, dirt is good[54] but if you look for specific benefits, probiotics are better.

Surge in Postbiotic Research

Postbiotics is a relatively new term that is gaining traction, especially since 2021 when the International Scientific Association for Probiotics and Prebiotics (ISAPP) published a consensus statement to propose a definition for the term: "postbiotics are a preparation of inanimate microorganisms and/or their components that confers a health benefit on the host."[55] However, this definition is polemic and challenged both by industry stakeholders and academics. The battle is still open for a definitive consensus.[56]

For example, Dr. Simone Guglielmetti from the University of Milan and speaker at Probiota 2022 challenges the conception that nonviable cells are mixed up in the same word with microbial factors, metabolites, and molecules emitted from these microorganisms. He proposes to call the dead cells "parabiotics" and the metabolites "postbiotics" (a distinction that has been used before,[57] and to avoid the term inanimate from this definition, which is not supported by the literature.[58] Indeed, you usually don't see live bacteria moving around on a Petri plate, so the notion that their livelihood should be identified through movement is questionable. The association avoided the commonly used term "inactive" to prevent risks of misinterpretation from the general public that "inactive microorganisms" would not exert activity and thus have health benefits. Implications are important for industry, regulators, and market trackers, who are waiting for a consistent rule to categorize these products in order to track their demand, success, and trends.

Interestingly, across different market sectors, as analyzed by consultant Luis Gosalbez, the term postbiotics refers to different realities: in food, it is mostly intended as inactivated (pasteurized or tyndallized) cells, whereas in cosmetics they imply lysates (cells broken into fragments) and in the drug segment, they describe isolated molecules.[59]

One of the reasons explaining the difficulty of reaching a consensus on the term is the challenge of isolating these different entities precisely and concretely in production. The manufacturing process for postbiotics includes fermentation, cleaning, and concentration of the biomass, and thereafter this cell-rich paste can be pasteurized to kill the cells. However, the end-product of this process will invariably include metabolites produced by the microorganisms, dead cells, as well as dead cells broken down in fragments.

Why is this Category Gaining Interest?

Well, the definition of probiotics implies that the microorganisms need to be alive. However, science has demonstrated that dead bacteria and their parts or metabolites can also exert health benefits, for example through the modulation of the immune system[60] and metabolic diseases[61] and this is of major importance to open the doors to pharmaceutical applications (it is much easier to apply for a drug status with an isolated molecule than with a live microorganism) and food applications (as live bacteria, as mentioned above, are sensitive to humidity, cooking, etc., and can't be included in foods or beverages that are processed in aggressive conditions or have a long shelf life).[62] For novel bacteria such as next-generation probiotics, a further implication is their safety: postbiotics may be superior in terms of safety relative to their mother cells. This is true for *Akkermansia muciniphila* which was granted the novel food status in Europe in 2021 only in its pasteurized form.[63] In this region, it will thus be a next-generation postbiotic.

CHAPTER 14

THERAPY TAKES UP A NOTCH WITH MICROBIOMES

As our knowledge about human microbiomes grows, one of the central ideas is its application in medicine. Basically, microbiomes can be used as therapy or we can use them to **complement** an existing therapy.

First, if microbiomes are to be used as **therapy**, important questions are:

1. What do we know about the links between the composition of a particular microbial community and a specific disease?
2. Which methods do we currently have available to manipulate microbiomes safely?
3. Which of these methods is best for a specific health condition?

In this chapter, we will address a few of the modern methods to manipulate microbiomes for therapy, such as microbial transplantation or phage therapy.

Second, if microbiomes are to be **combined** to improve the outcome of another therapy, we need to know their mutual interactions. A special branch of microbiome science, popularly called "pharmacomicrobiomics" is addressing the question of microbiome-drug interactions.

Finally, as each patient is unique in their genetic background, hormonal status, etc., but also their microbiome composition, the imperative for successful therapy is to be *personalized.*

Various Microbial Transplantation Therapies

In the ancient Chinese book titled *Zhou Hou Bei Ji Fang* written about 1,700 years ago (translated as "Handbook of Emergency Medicine"), traditional Chinese medicine doctor Ge Hong, among other methods, described the use of "yellow soup" (actually, human stool preparation!) as a treatment against food poisoning and severe diarrhea. Legend also says that some Bedouin tribes used to eat the feces of their camels as a remedy for gut problems. Later reports from the 18th, 19th, and 20th centuries described the use of stool preparation on soldiers affected by dysentery (gut infection caused by *Shigella* or amoebae). Anyway, a study published in 1958 by American Surgeon Dr. Ben Eisenmann and colleagues, describing the successful recovery of four patients from bacterial gut infection (Enterocolitis) treated by rectal application of stool suspension from a healthy donor, is considered an official beginning of modern Fecal Microbiome Transplant—also known as FMT therapy.[1]

We previously discussed what a healthy microbiome actually is, and mentioned that a small percentage of healthy people might have bacterial species in their gut, which are typically associated with serious infections. One such example is *Clostridioides difficile* Infection (CDI), a life-threatening diarrhea triggered by gut dysbiosis (for example, by overuse of antibiotics). AN important feature of CDI, as in many other bacterial infections, is that a single bacterial species outcompetes other species. Obviously, this situation can be restored by providing fresh bacterial communities, for example, from the fecal material of a healthy door. CDI is currently the most common indication for the application of FMT.[2] As we learned in Part III, gut dysbiosis is the root of, not only of the gut but various other health conditions. Therefore, CDI is certainly not the only possible application of FMT. The spectrum is large—from gastric conditions such as Irritable Bowel Disorder, Ulcerative Colitis, or liver disease to non-gastric problems, such as metabolic diseases, allergies, neurological, skin, and support to cancer immunotherapy.[3] There are specialized clinics around the world where FMT therapy can be performed. So far, nine biobanks are storing fecal samples of healthy donors for prospective patients. Legal guidelines exist currently only for CDI but hundreds of clinical studies are underway.[4] However, some important issues are still to be improved. The procedure itself, from the sample preparation, rigorous quality control, and selection of donors, to the sophistication of the delivery methods. From the ancient Chinese "yellow soup," oral and rectal delivery, we advanced to the simple oral capsules. Future directions will likely include well-defined microbial consortia and personalized solutions. In fact, SER-109, the first clinically approved microbiome-based drug (made by company Seres Therapeutics for therapy of recurrent CDI), was created by purification of 50 specific bacterial species selected from the donor stool.[5]

Similar to the gut, dysbiosis can happen elsewhere in the organism. We have mentioned Bacterial Vaginosis (BV) before, a condition characterized by the decrease in the Lactobacilli and an increase in other bacterial species. Typical treatments for BV are either antibiotics or probiotics. As usual, the problem with antibiotics is that it causes a further decrease in bacterial diversity and frequent recurrence of the infection. The problem with probiotics is that only a limited number of species have been registered on the market and, although they could improve the condition, they do not restore natural diversity. Therefore, Vaginal Microbiome Transplantation (also known as VMT) seems as a promising option. Similar to FMT, samples for VMT are isolated from the vaginal secretion of healthy donors, quality-checked, and transferred into the vagina of a patient. Initial VMT clinical trials have shown significant improvements in BV patients.[6] Except for BV, another area of VMT application is "seeding" babies born by Cesarean section by the mother's vaginal microbiome, which can have great health benefits, as previously discussed.

Human skin is the next emerging area of microbiome-transplantation therapy. Skin conditions such as atopic dermatitis or acne are also examples of bacterial dysbiosis. Future research will have to determine whether transplanting whole microbiomes of a particular skin area or the application of a well-defined microbial mixture will provide better clinical results.[7]

Human microbiomes are dynamic communities, changing with food intake, lifestyle, etc. Therefore, the stability and long-term duration of the microbiome transplantation therapy pose a challenge. Another concern is that our current microbial transplants are mainly based on bacteria and, to have a complete picture we would need to learn more about the roles of viruses, fungi, and protozoans in the complexity of human microbiomes.

Phage Therapy

It was the year 1933 in Tbilisi, Georgia, Soviet Union. Felix d'Herelle, the scientist who discovered bacteriophages (viruses that infect and can kill bacteria), came to visit his colleague George Eliava at the Institute for Bacteriophage Therapy. Actually, it was the first institute in the world dedicated to bacteriophage therapy, founded by Eliava and inspired by the works of d'Herelle. Unfortunately, the great scientific collaboration didn't last long. Eliava made a cardinal mistake by falling in love with the same woman as Lavrenti Beria, chief of the Soviet secret service, NKVD (later known as KGB). Long story short, in 1937 Eliava was declared "people's enemy" and shot dead. Felix d'Herelle had to leave Georgia but the institute continued working and does so until the present day.[8]

Some years later, during the Cold War, the western world was delighted by the use of penicillin against bacterial infections and nobody really thought about bacteriophages as potential antimicrobial agents. Paradoxically, however, in the same western world, bacteriophages were the key that demonstrated that DNA, and not proteins, is the hereditary material and were responsible for several other seminal discoveries and Nobel Prizes in molecular biology. But nobody in the west used them as anti-infective therapy for humans.

This is what happens when politics interferes with science. A story rather good for a movie?

A few decades after the Cold War, our arsenal of antibacterial weapons is getting thinner and thinner. Multiresistant bacterial strains which no antibiotic can kill are becoming more rule than the exception. Suddenly, politics is not so important anymore and the interest in bacteriophages, or so-called "phage therapy" is rising again globally. In the United States, several companies such as Intralytix, BioMx, Adaptive Phage Therapeutics, or PhagePro, are focused on applications of phages for therapies and food safety. In Europe, there are a couple of phage companies such as Phagomed or Lysando, but there is still a lag due to the non-existent regulatory framework, with the companies mostly focused on products without living phages (e.g. phage Lysins).

Let's note that bacteriophages are tiny, but the most numerous organisms on our planet (estimates are 10^31!). They are everywhere: in the oceans, on land, in all living things, and wherever there are bacteria. So far, more than 140,000 unique phages have been identified in the human gut.[9] Scientists are currently building special databases for phage genomes. We are approaching an exciting future where, ideally, for each pathogenic bacteria we will be able to isolate at least several different phages as an anti-bacterial option. Furthermore, soon we might be able to selectively target desired bacteria and modify our microbiomes.

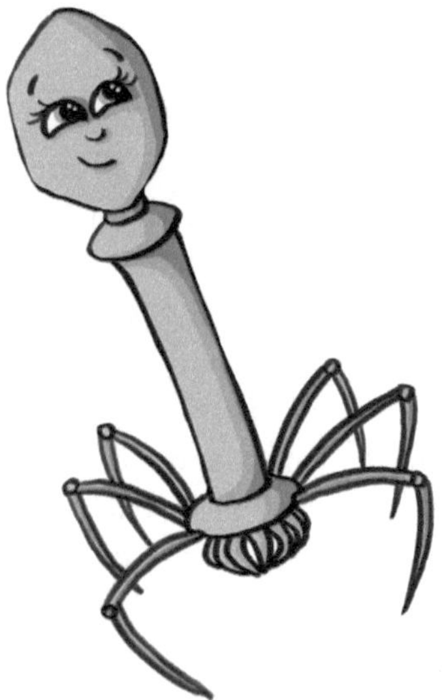

Fig. 14.1 Bacteriophages are bacterial viruses which were key for several crucial discoveries in molecular biology. They are again gaining importance in microbiome-based therapies.

Pharmacomicrobiomics

Our gut microbiota is involved in various activities like metabolizing food, synthesis of vitamins, immune functions, etc.[10] It is therefore not a surprise that the gut microbiota influences the way xenobiotics or drugs are metabolized. Enter the newly coined term—pharmaco-microbiomics. Put simply, pharmacomicrobiomics is a new field that studies drug–microbiome interactions. Specifically, this field tries to study and understand the intra- and inter-individual microbiome variations affecting drug action, disposition, efficacy, and toxicity.[11]

Many factors play a role in the efficacy of a drug including age, genetics, disease, etc.[12] Recent evidence suggests that gut microbiota may too contribute as to how a drug is metabolized and hence made available to the host.[13] Not only this, the gut microbiota has a bidirectional interaction with the drugs. Gut microbiota influences drug availability and drugs might also affect the composition of the gut microbiota.

A. Drugs Affecting the Microbiota Composition

Drugs once orally ingested pass through the upper gastrointestinal tract to the small intestine and finally to the colon where they encounter the various microbial species. Drugs can alter the metabolism of the microbes, modify the intestinal environment or directly affect the growth of the microbes thereby influencing microbial community composition and function. Let's look at some of the research with regard to how the drugs influence gut microbiota composition. Antibiotics are prescribed to treat bacterial infections. These compounds have been shown to disrupt the normal microbiota ecosystem of the intestine.[14]Not only antibiotics but in a recent study, it was found that some anti-cancer drugs such as daunorubicin, 5-fluorouracil, floxuridine, and even anti-rheumatic drug, auranofin, were toxic to certain bacteria in the gut, highlighting how these drugs might change the intestinal microbiome profile of the patients consuming these drugs.[15] Interestingly, it was found that proton pump inhibitors (prescribed for treating acid reflux or gastroesophageal reflux disease—GERD) had the biggest effect on the gut microbiome, similar in effect to antibiotics.[16] But not all drugs impact the gut microbiota negatively. It has been proposed that metformin, a drug commonly prescribed to treat type 2 diabetes may show its therapeutic effect by increasing the abundance of the beneficial gut bacterium *Akkermansia muciniphila*.[17]

B. Microbiota Affecting the Drugs

There are multiple ways by which the microbiota in the gut may affect the drugs. They may influence their efficacy, availability, toxicity, etc (Fig. 14.2). Let's look at some of these effects:

Microbiota effect on drug activity:

Sulfasalazine, a drug used in the treatment of ulcerative colitis, gets activated in the gut by the bacterial cleavage of azo bonds leading to site-specific release of sulfapyridine and 5-aminosalicylic acid- both having anti-inflammatory effects.[18] Microbial transformation of the drugs might lower their activity too. Digoxin, a cardiovascular drug gets reduced by specific *Eggarthella lenta* strains thereby rendering it inactive.[19]

Microbiota effect on drug toxicity:

The toxicity of drugs happens when microbial transformations produce metabolites that negatively affect the host. One of the best-known examples in this aspect is the colon cancer drug, Irinotecan. Irinotecan can cause severe diarrhea in many patients. The active metabolite of the drug gets glucuronidated in the liver to its inactive form. It has been shown that bacterial beta-glucuronidases reactivate the drug in the intestine causing toxicity toward the intestinal epithelial cells, leading to diarrhea.

Microbiota effect on drug availability:

L-Dopa or levodopa is the drug given for the treatment of Parkinson's disease. However, the bioavailability of L-Dopa varies significantly among Parkinson's disease patients. One of the reasons for the variable bioavailability of this drug is due to the conversion of L-Dopa to dopamine by the bacteria in the intestine.[20] Patients with a higher abundance of *Enterococcus faecalis* might be converting L-Dopa to dopamine before it can cross the blood-brain barrier thereby reducing the drug's bioavailability.

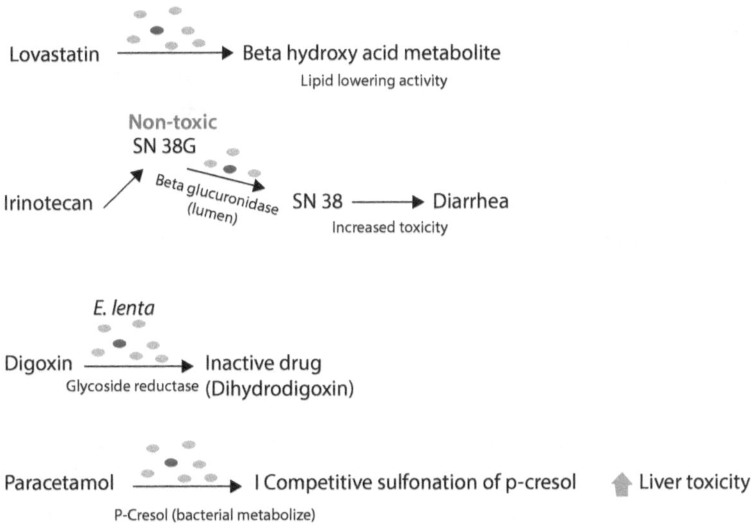

Fig. 14.2   Ways in which gut microbiota modulate drugs

Microbiota effect on modulating clinical response:

Immuno-checkpoint inhibitors such as PD-1 inhibitors and CTLA-4 inhibitors are a new class of anti-cancer drugs that work by allowing the T-cells (a kind of immune cells) to kill the cancer cells. However, the overall response rate to these drugs varies and is 20–40 percent.[21] Several reports now have shown that patients responding to immune-checkpoint inhibitors have a different gut microbiota profile as compared to the non-responders.[22] A higher bacterial diversity and the presence of "good" bacteria such as *Akkermansia muciniphila* were found in the responders.[23]

C. Pharmacomicrobiomics—Importance and Future Potential

Inter-individual response to drugs varies and can cause variable efficacy and toxicity. Adverse drug reactions and lower efficacy not only can negatively affect individual wellbeing but also posts a tremendous financial burden. It is estimated that in the United States alone, serious drug toxicities cause over 100,000 deaths and cost over 30 billion dollars annually.[24] Therefore, we need a fresh understanding of how drugs affect us. With the advent of new technologies like next-generation sequencing and new culturing methods, we are now beginning to delve better into the world of microbiota. With the knowledge of how microbiota in the gut affect drugs we can synthesize and develop:

1.   Drugs that are more efficacious
2.   Drugs that are less toxic
3.   Improve drug availability

All the above will lead to an era of personalized medicine in the true sense. For example, once we know that a particular bacterium is needed to activate a drug and if the bacteria is less abundant in a patient, we can deliver the bacteria along with the drug during the course of the treatment to improve its effectiveness. Similarly, we can screen people based on their gut microbiota profile before starting chemotherapeutic treatment so that the chances of success are high which will lead to better economics and improved quality of life for cancer patients. Another very important aspect that needs attention is nutrition. Certain nutrients are known to promote or decrease specific microbes. *E. lenta* inactivates digoxin and is inhibited by dietary arginine.[25] Finally, the present technologies that help profile gut microbiota should be encouraged more, especially in the clinical setting to help health professionals take an informed decision on the best course of action for their patients!

To What Extent Therapy can be Personalized?

Personalized medicine is the newly emerging field of medicine, considered by many experts as the future of medicine in general. The idea behind the personalized approach is that a therapy is adapted to each patient according to various individual genetic, physiological, and other parameters, with a goal of lowering the risks and increasing positive responses to the therapy.

A good example of how human microbiomes can be used in personalized therapy approach is the above-mentioned modulation of the clinical response to cancer immunotherapy. Overall bacterial richness, as well as the presence of specific bacteria, has been measured for several different immune checkpoint inhibitors (ICIs) and different types of tumors.[26] More studies are currently ongoing to determine the mechanisms of the microbial effects in ICI and eventual applications in other types of immunotherapy. These mechanisms could, for example, involve the production of microbial compounds toxic to cancer cells, stimulation of the immune system (see chapter about the microbiome and immune system), modulation of drug metabolism (see above), or a combination thereof. As this area is also commercially very attractive, several companies such as 4D-Pharma, Microbiotica, Prokarium, Second Genome, Everimmune, Da Volterra or Enterome, are already exploring living bacteria, small molecules, or peptides, as therapeutics to be combined with ICIs or other types of cancer therapies, such as radio- or chemotherapy.

Biomarkers and microbial signatures (which we will discuss in the next chapter), can be used to predict the therapy outcome and personalize the approach, not only for cancer therapy but also for other conditions.

The Journey of Discovering a New Drug

Drug discovery is a long and expensive process. Government bodies and pharmaceutical companies invest tens of billions of dollars every year on it. Typically, the first step in the process is the identification of a potential target, for example, a molecule involved in the mechanisms of disease. The next step is the screening of a large number of components, predicted to hit the selected target, by a series of assays. Best candidates, also known as "drug leads," are then selected and further tested for their activity against the target, eventual toxic effects, etc. Selected leads are then used for further drug development and eventually in clinical trials.[27]

Throughout the book, we have learned that the members of our microbiomes produce components that influence our organs and organ systems directly or by stimulating our cells, such as the gut, nerve, or immune cells, to produce molecules with physiological effects in our body. In this sense, our microbes already work as drugs. In the chapters about probiotics and microbial transplantation therapy, we discussed the possibilities of using living microbes as therapeutics (alone or in mixtures, e.g bacterial consortia). In the parts about personalized therapy and pharmacomicrobiomics we discussed how microbes can influence existing drugs and therapies.

Another opportunity to use microbiomes is to identify and extract bioactive compounds synthesized by microbes. These could be peptides or small molecules, such as short-chain fatty acids, amino acids, neurotransmitters, or many others, yet unknown molecules. However, the spectrum of microbially-produced, physiologically active components is not limited only to human microbiomes. Other microbes are everywhere, living with other organisms and freely in the environment.

Around 50 percent of all our drugs come directly from natural (or biological) sources or are based on them. Others are partially or fully chemically synthesized, using natural molecules (or their parts) as examples, or by modifying existing drugs. Literally, one drug (or maybe two) available on the market has been synthesized using only combinatorial chemistry.[28] Another point, all vaccines and most of the antibiotics we have come from microorganisms, as well as more than 120 most important drugs.[29] In part 1, we mentioned that by using our traditional microbiological methods, we were able to grow only around 1 percent of all existing microorganisms. Microbiome research is opening a possibility to explore other 99 percent microbes as a potential source of new drugs.

A great example in this area is the United States-based company Biosortia Microbiomics. Using their innovative technology, it became possible to extract microbiomes from thousands of liters of water within a couple of hours, creating libraries of small molecules. Other important technologies empowering microbiome-based drug discovery are the "omics" technologies, such as metagenomics, proteomics, and metabolomics. Artificial intelligence, in particular machine-learning algorithms, can accelerate the discovery of the best drug leads by processing huge amounts of data.[30] In the near future, we expect to see the development of more libraries and databases of microbiome-relevant small molecules and informatics tools for their analysis.

CHAPTER 15

MICROBIOMES CAN EVEN DIAGNOSE DISEASES

THE Covid-19 pandemic made the use of the word biomarkers quite colloquial. Often heard in the media, biomarker is a term mostly used in clinical studies or when people talk about diagnostics.

Here is what US Food and Drug Administration (FDA) says about it:

"*Biomarker* is a defined characteristic that is measured as an indicator of normal biological processes, pathogenic processes, or responses to an exposure or intervention, including therapeutic interventions."

There are different categories of biomarkers. Those which can diagnose a disease, predict a disease and its outcome or a response to a particular therapy, determine the toxicity of a substance, etc.[1]

If we think about a microbial disease, any microbial species can be regarded as a diagnostic biomarker. For example, if we find *Mycobacterium tuberculosis* in a patient who has symptoms of tuberculosis, we can say with a high probability that he or she has the disease. Also, a bacterial protein or a toxin can be used as a biomarker: if a Shiga-Toxin is detected in the stool of a patient with the symptoms of food poisoning, it is most likely caused by an enteropathogenic strain of the bacterium *Escherichia coli*.

With the advancement of microbiome research, there has been growing interest in finding microbial biomarkers for health, disease prevention, and diagnostics of various conditions, which were discussed in Part 3. We already learned that ratios between certain types (taxa) of gut microbes (e.g. Firmicutes, Bacteroidetes), or the presence of probiotic ones (*Bifidobacterium*, *Lactobacillus*, *Akkermansia*, etc.) can serve as biomarkers for our general health and, as guidelines for personalized nutrition. As we will see in the next chapters, this possibility has been already exploited by several companies.

A fresh example of microbial biomarkers linked to the prevention and outcome of a disease is COVID-19. It has been shown that monitoring gut and lung microbiota can help to predict the severity of the disease and, possibly serve as a way to select the right probiotics for the prevention of so-called "long-COVID".[2] Second, bacteria are also biomarkers for risk and prognosis in some cancer types. Typical examples include *Helicobacter pylori* and gastric cancers or *Fusobacterium nucleatum* and colorectal cancer.[3] *Fusobacterium* has been often found in high numbers in stool samples of patients with severe disease progression, poor prognosis, and therapy outcome.[4] Other studies evaluated bacteria or their metabolites as diagnostic and prognostic biomarkers for gastrointestinal conditions (e.g. Crohn's disease, ulcerative colitis, inflammatory bowel disease [IBD]),[5] or neurological conditions (Alzheimer's disease, Parkinson's disease, schizophrenia, and autism).[6] In Chapter 16, we will discuss the roles of microbiomes in cancer therapy. Recent research data has shown that the success of immune checkpoint inhibitor (ICI) therapy for various cancer types is linked to the individual composition of a patient's gut microbiomes. Several potential biomarkers have been already identified as predictors of ICI therapy response.[7]

Besides the usual cancer diagnostic of tumor markers in the blood, detection of circulating microbial biomarkers from different body fluids (so-called "liquid biopsy"), seems to be a promising diagnostics alternative.[8] The company, Karius Health is a pioneering example of liquid biopsy applications for diagnostics of various microbial pathogens.

Microbial Signatures: Defining the Biomarkers can be Tricky

Sometimes a disease or a condition may be caused or linked to multiple microbes. For instance, interactions can happen between bacterial strains (a level below species), different microbial species, or higher taxonomic categories (families, genera, etc.). It could also be that only particular genes, proteins, or metabolites (produced by completely different microbes) are important. Therefore, instead of biomarker, the term "microbial signature" is used. A microbial signature is defined as a "set of interacting biomarkers, and the relationship that they have with the host phenotype."[9]

With an increasing set of parameters, the number of possible combinations for interactions in microbial signatures is enormous. To decipher these, scientists are using various approaches, such as previously mentioned machine-learning methods. For example, a set of features linked to the particular composition of a microbial community can be used to train the program.[10] So far, microbial signatures have been used to diagnose IBD, Crohn's disease, obesity, and diabetes. Linking microbial signatures and drug metabolism have been proposed for breast cancers.[11] Another successful fresh example is the FDA-approved test for oral cancer by the company, Viome.[12]

Thrilling World of Forensics

Another interesting application of microbiome biomarkers is in forensic science. At the start of this book, we learned that the composition of microbial populations differs among our body sites. This can be used to determine microbiome traces on different objects or body parts. For example, microbial signatures from pubic hair can determine if a person was a victim of a sexual assault. Other forensic uses of human microbiomes help identification of a person, time after death, manner and cause of death or, based on the presence of other microbiomes (soil, other animals, etc.), to link a person with a location.[13]

With the technical advancements and increase in biological knowledge (for example, amounts of data for training of machine-learning algorithms), there is a high probability that we will be soon able to routinely apply microbiome-based biomarkers, alone or combined with the traditional diagnostic methods, for early detection and prevention of the diseases, adjustment of individual therapies, in forensics and other fields.

An important field where microbiota can indicate a shift between a healthy or a diseased state is certainly human nutrition, details of which we will discuss in the following chapter.

CHAPTER 16

CHOOSING NUTRITION WISELY!

> "Let food be thy medicine and medicine be thy food."
>
> —Hippocrates

MOST human cultures, traditions, or religions, involve certain kinds of habits and practices regarding periods of fasting or avoiding certain types of food. Since ancient times, people have known the effects of nutrition on our physical and mental well-being. In Part III, we discussed the concept of a "healthy microbiome" and its systemic effects on our bodies, for which there is solid evidence of links to the composition of our gut microbiomes. Every time we eat, trillions of invisible "assistants" in our guts help our digestion. To understand how they exactly do this, we need to look closer into the composition of our food.

Speaking in the language of biochemistry, our food essentially consists of three main categories of nutrient molecules: sugars (carbohydrates), proteins, and fats. Sugars can be further divided into two types: those that our body can easily digest and those which cannot. For example, simple sugars from fruits or milk, belong to the first one. More complex, digestion-resistant starches and plant fibers are examples of the second type. As discussed in Chapter 7, consuming more of one of another type of carbohydrate determines which type of bacteria will grow in our gut "garden." Having too much of one kind (Firmicutes) can make us fatter or even obese, and too much of another (Bacteroidetes) slimmer. In the chapter about prebiotics, we also mentioned that hard-to-digest plant fibers are good food for our beneficial gut microbes.

Let's Understand Various Compounds from the Food We Eat!

Cellulose is the most abundant biological molecule on our planet, present in all plants and therefore also in all of our plant-based food. Cells of our body are not able to chemically break down this complex sugar-polymer and it reaches our gut mostly in the form of insoluble fibers. These fibers have a fantastic ability to absorb lots of water, thus increasing in volume and, by giving gentle "pinpricks" to our gut walls, stimulating their movements. Without these movements, it would be very hard, if not impossible, to complete the digestive process and get rid of the food-rests from our guts. Except for the mechanical role, another great thing about plant fibers is that they are the favorite food for some of our gut microbes. These microbes possess a special degrading enzyme (e.g. cellulase), degrading complex sugar polymers into simpler sugars that can be used then as an energy source. A stark difference, however, is that oxygen, normally used for the burning of sugars in the cells (glycolysis), is not readily available in the gut. Therefore, a type of product from this process (also known as fermentation) are smaller molecules, such as short-chain fatty acids (SCFAs). In recent years, various beneficial effects of SCFAs on the human body have been shown—from regulating appetite and improving sugar metabolism (such as in obese people) to regulating blood pressure, and strengthening gut walls (gut-blood barrier), thus preventing undesired molecules to reach our bloodstream and boosting our immunity.[1] The effect of other dietary fibers and their effect on the human microbiome is an intense field of research.

On the other side, a high-fat diet changes the composition of the gut microbiome, so that SCFAs and beneficial Bifidobacteria lessen while Bacteroidetes increase.[2] Various types of fats are also important. In general, saturated fats (especially trans-saturated) have been shown to increase inflammation in mice and vice versa. Certain types of polyunsaturated fats have been shown to have beneficial effects on the gut microbiome, reducing inflammation.[3] Effects of a special diet consisting of high fat and low carbohydrates (aka Keto diet) have anti-inflammatory effects in obese people. However, the Keto diet is known to bear potential health risks.[4]

Proteins from the food are enzymatically digested to peptides and amino acids in the small intestine by proteases and peptidases. Relatively recently, we learned that microbiomes of the small intestine, as well as large intestine and colon, are also involved in this process. Depending on the type or source of a protein (e.g. plant or animal), gut microbes can digest or transform proteins into different metabolites such as SCFAs, (bad-smelling) hydrogen sulfide, polyamines, ammonia, phenols, indoles, and others. These metabolites can influence various processes in the body. The availability of particular proteins or amino acids from the food influences the composition of the gut microbiome. Very high protein or very low protein diet can have negative effects on the gut microbiome, stimulating the growth of potentially pathogenic bacteria or decreasing probiotics ones respectively.[5]

Sauerkraut, kimchi, yogurt, kombucha, pickles, and similar fermented food are known as great sources of probiotic strain, such as yeasts (Saccharomyces), Lactobaccili, and Bifidobacteria. Vitamins, such as B-complex, are directly produced by some gut bacteria. Food supplementation with Vitamins A, C, D, and E modulates or increases several probiotic gut bacteria.

Regarding other non-nutrient food compounds, it is worth mentioning polyphenols, which increase the abundance of beneficial bacteria (e.g. Bifidobacteria) and decrease potentially pathogenic ones (e.g. Clostridium species). Typical polyphenol-rich foods are berries, seeds, some vegetables, cocoa (e.g dark chocolate), and wine. On the other side, (as mentioned in the part about weight management), betaines and choline from animal-based food could have potentially negative effects by being converted into trimethylamine (TMA) by gut microbes and finally into TMA-N-Oxide (TMAO) in the liver. TMAO has been linked with pro-inflammatory processes (e.g. in obesity and cardiometabolic diseases) and carcinogenesis.[6] This list is certainly not exhaustive. There are various non-dietary food compounds, such as additives, pollutants, etc., for which the interactions with the microbiome are being studied. During the last decades, there has been a rapid increase in the consumption of processed, simple sugars, saturated fats, food additives, preservatives, antibiotics, and pollutants in a typical western diet. In parallel with that, we witness a surge in various health conditions, many of which are listed throughout this book. A large part of the current microbiome research is focused on finding possible connections between our microbiomes and our nutrition.

Scientific advances not only in the microbiome field but also in human genomics and physiology have opened new possibilities for individually tailored dietary advice, a new booming field, sometimes called "Precision Nutrition." Many companies and entrepreneurs have realized the potential, not only for therapeutic applications but also for a global consumer market. Currently, there are dozens of companies offering gut-microbiome analytics, based on which nutritional advice is provided. There is a difference between their methodology and the scope of the services. Some companies provide traditional, cultivation-based microbiological analytics, others sequence DNA by next-generation sequencing (see Part II about sequencing), detecting the microbes down to the species or even strain level. The United States-based company Viome went even further, analyzing RNA (expressed genes). Other companies, such as Metabolome, Enzymetrix, or Biocrates are focused on the analysis of metabolic products of microbiomes. Deciding exactly which kind of analysis to do depends largely on which kind of information we need such as specific gut illness, potential pathogens, general gut health, microbiome diversity, or the presence of beneficial bacteria.[7] Some companies provide complete packages, including food supplements, dietary, wellness or fitness plans, blood, metabolic or other kinds of analysis. This is often combined with a modern data output format using, for example, mobile apps for health tracking and data collection.

Breaking It Down

The concept of personalized nutrition comes from the observation that different people have different nutritional needs. Beyond people with medical conditions whose needs are covered by foods developed especially for them, called foods for special medical purposes, you and I, even if we have the same age, gender, and level of physical activity, can react very differently to different foods.

The premises of this sector came with human genome sequencing. The huge project started in 1988 and was (partially) completed 15 years after, on 14 April 2003.[8] It offered humankind the awareness that although we have the same amounts of genes, about 23,000, we don't carry the same genes in the same amounts. This is relevant in nutrition. For example, if you do not present genes producing lactase, the enzyme degrading lactose, you are more likely to be lactose intolerant. More likely, not certainly lactose intolerant, because you may harbor bacteria in your microbiota that produce lactase and help you with lactose digestion. Certain companies, like DNAFit or Genomelink,[9] provide dietary personalized recommendations based on genome analysis and lifestyle questionnaires, especially taking into account micronutrient needs such as vitamins.

The next level of personalized nutrition is based on even more information and includes gut microbiota analysis. Because our food gets to our microbes before it gets absorbed in our bloodstream, we need to consider the interaction with microbes for a full picture of what's going on. Israeli company DayTwo[10] is a pioneer in this sector. They collect information on the microbiome, blood tests, questionnaires, anthropometrics, and a food diary, then the information is churned and ground by artificial intelligence and a machine learning algorithm based on strong science,[11] the company provides recommendations on which foods will provoke a glycemia peak in a given individual, and in which combinations they can be less damageable. The fascinating aspect of this work is that common sense about foods with a high glycemic index (white bread, muffins, cookies, etc.) are turned upside down. For some people, a cookie may be a better option than a banana, from the point of view of glycemia. The Weizmann Institute researchers saw that some people's blood sugar spiked more after eating sushi than after eating ice cream, questioning the foundation of the universal nature of healthy foods.[12]

These results are exciting because DayTwo's personalized recommendations are not only easier to follow for people, they are superior to the standard of care in neutralizing the blood sugar response to food and are already helping people manage and prevent diabetes through their diet.

There are Loopholes!

Although these results are powerful and exciting, I would like to stress a limitation inherent to the concept of personalized nutrition. Families struggle to find the time to cook fresh produce every day for the whole family. Cooking for each separate individual in the family would become a tremendous, if not impossible, chore. The risk, with taking different meals, is to buy ready-meals from the groceries and warm them up in single portions. This would imply an increase in processed and ultra-processed foods, and likely as well a reduction in the diversity of meals. Both aspects have shown associations with negative health outcomes including overweight, obesity, cardio-metabolic risks, cancer, type-2 diabetes, cancer, irritable bowel syndrome, and even all-cause mortality.[13]

Another limitation of personalized nutrition regards another role that food plays in human life: conviviality. The pleasure of eating together the same meal at the same table, freshly prepared, is an overlooked player in mental and physical wellness. As of yet, as an agronomy engineer with a nutrition specialization, I am not convinced that the health benefits of extreme personalization would outweigh the drawbacks. This being said, a better awareness of each of the family member's own specificities and needs can help make better choices while keeping a fresh, inclusive meal on the table.

Testing Your Gut at Home

The next level of personalized nutrition is based on even more information and includes gut microbiota analysis. Since our food gets to our microbes before it gets absorbed in our bloodstream, we need to consider the interaction with microbes for a full picture of what's going on.

It all began in 2012 when a non-profit, American Gut Project established a data collection platform, in order to supply the necessary research to allow the field to thrive. Today, more and more companies are offering their own microbiome services, in one form or another—and the count continues. In Europe, GUTXY was the first microbiome testing company in Denmark. They introduced mainstream use of dietary interventions with microbiome testing, thanks to their RESET+ program that allows individuals to test their diet before and after they test their gut. In this way, people can track how their gut microbes react to the consumption of different foods. Meanwhile, DayTwo focuses on the microbiome in combination with glycemic responses.[14] They've demonstrated that individual blood sugar responses can be surprising—such as ice cream performing better than sushi for some people.

Every trend has its early adopters and, when it comes to microbiome testing, they often have a fascination with fitness and optimizing their health. They want to give themselves an edge, feel better, and they believe that understanding more about the community that lives inside them will do just that. On the other hand, others discover microbiome testing due to personal needs. In the United States alone,

62 million Americans are diagnosed with a digestive disorder every year.[15] Even without a diagnosis, everyone would have experienced a digestive symptom in their lifetime: bloating, constipation, and diarrhea. In those where it's prevalent, this can create a psychological and emotional burden.

What we've learned through microbiome research has affirmed what we've always wondered: your health is a summary of your lineage, daily habits, and environment. Our genetics have been emphasized, but they are something that is largely out of our control. That's the beauty of our microbiome: it's malleable. How we eat and live on a daily basis directly impacts our gut composition.

Our microbes sculpt our organs, break down our food, help us defend against infections and even guide our behavior. By studying and understanding our microbiomes, we've been able to highlight their importance. These microbial cells outnumber our human ones.[16] So far, we have named only a fraction of these microbes, and even substantially less have noted functional information. We know they're there, but we don't know why or what purpose they're serving. Naturally, this can create confusion.

Some microbes are better known than others. *Lactobacillus* and *Bifidobacteria* have been researched to exhaustion (given how easy they are to cash in on as commercial probiotics.) Meanwhile, other microbes have proven to provide beneficial effects when supported through a microbiome-friendly diet, such as *Akkermansia muciniphila*, *Fecalibacterium prauznitzii*, and *Roseburia*.

The Power of Microbiome Testing

Ultimately, microbiome testing lets you see a world you wouldn't have otherwise. You get to see how diverse your gut is, and which microbes are living with you.

You can only learn about what microbes are inside you by testing them. It is that simple: if you believe your gut microbes matter for your health, and want to know how healthy your gut is, test it!

However, be forewarned: testing can reveal a lot of information. The process can seem more like a mystery than a solution. A long list of Latin names for different bacteria can be overwhelming for the average person. It gets even tricky when you want to know what number you should have.

No microbiome test can tell you: the difference between a red or green apple, the exact amounts you should be eating, or what all your microbes are specifically doing. The data is too vast.

What microbiome testing can give you is:

- Your gut's unique microbial composition at the time of sampling
- Information about whether these microbes are associated with health or disease
- Suggestions for increasing or decreasing certain microbes
- Interpretations of your results using the most recent scientific literature

Your microbiome is a maze. The more we learn, the more we realize what we don't know. This is as much a chicken-and-egg game as it is a time-sensitive soup. Fortunately, thousands of researchers are dedicated to understanding the microbiome.

Microbiome science is constantly evolving. Knowing what your microbiome looks like today, can give you insights to use for your future.

The Need for Better Sampling Standards

Current stool sampling techniques could be improved. Of course, fresher samples are preferred. However, most people don't want to freeze their poop or have the time to take it to the lab right away. As discussed in Chapter 2, that's why stabilization solutions are typically put in place. This gives the sample time to be shipped to the lab, whilst still preserving the valuable microbial data.

However, researchers in different labs are typically working with different tubes, solutions, and lab protocols. Reproducibility requires a similar set of measures, making it more difficult to compare samples and data from different labs.

Thus, with no "golden" lab standard, we can be left to debate on what methodology is better. This can slow growth. Standardization of sampling and testing methods is key to moving the field further.

CHAPTER 17

THEY ARE IN YOUR EVERYDAY PRODUCTS!

Beyond nutritional advice and gut-microbiome testing, there are other areas where non-clinical, microbiome-based products and services are already available for general consumers.

Cosmetic skin care is certainly one of the promising segments in this fast-growing market. Large cosmetics companies are already catching the wave: for example, Nivea claims that its products are keeping the skin microbiome "in balance", Vichy (Loreal) recently launched its first anti-dandruff shampoo, Lancome (Loreal) its skin anti-aging lotion with a mixture of probiotics and prebiotics. Companies such as Clearskin, VGAM, Dermala, Cybelemicrobiome, Gladskin, Vemico, Mother Dirt, Gallinee, and others, are providing food supplements (prebiotics) or live bacterial strains (probiotics), which, when taken orally or applied directly on the skin as creams, oils, sprays, soap bars, body washes and similar, are reported to have rejuvenating or anti-aging effects, reducing wrinkles, moistening skin or making it shinier and elastic. Creams and lotions with microorganisms supporting sun protection or preventing hair loss will probably be soon in the new product lines. Company Givaudan launched a skin-microbiome-friendly fragrance (Z-Biome). Similar to gut-microbiome testing, skin-microbiome sampling and sequencing are now also available, often combined with genetic or other kinds of analysis, personalized advice, and personalized cosmetic products. Examples include Dr. Elsa Jungman or Sequential Skin.

Human sweat is colorless and odorless fluid. However, metabolites produced by the skin microbiome are mostly those responsible for our body odors. We already learned that reducing microbial richness and diversity by application of antimicrobial substances on any body part is generally not a good idea. The same is valid for our skin. For example, commonly used antiperspirants have been shown to decrease microbial richness and stimulate the growth of microbes responsible for bad odor.

Scientist Dave Whitlock, the founder of the company AOBiome, seems to be someone who takes care of his skin-microbiome very seriously. Allegedly he didn't shower for the last twelve years, only applying beneficial, ammonia-oxidizing bacteria (sold also by his company), on his skin. We don't know whether this is true or not, but people around him say he doesn't smell bad and is mostly in a good mood.

Talking about body odors, most of us have experienced the unpleasant situation of somebody's bad breath. Again, in most of these cases, little microbial companions in our mouths are to blame and not because of eating too much garlic or onion. The older concept of maintaining oral hygiene by killing microbes with chlorine-based or similar antibacterial mouthwashes is fading away and we have realized that the richness and diversity of oral microbiomes are crucial, not only for good breath but also for our oral and general health. A recent example is a collaboration between the microbiome data-science company Eagle Genomics and the global consumer goods company Unilever, resulting in microbiome-based toothpaste (ZendiumTM) which selectively increases beneficial oral microbes, while it decreases harmful ones.[1]

As our knowledge about oral bacteria grows, we will probably see more consumer products based on probiotic oral bacteria. For example, strains of *Streptococcus salivarius*, a beneficial bacterium, found in human saliva are found in probiotic bombons or chewing gums of the company called Blis Probiotics. Previous studies have shown that *S. salivarius* reduces risk of *Streptococcus mutans*, bacterium known to cause dental caries.

In Chapter 10, we discussed the importance of the microbiome for female urogenital health and the harmful effects of removal of beneficial vaginal bacteria and yeast. Consumer products for female intimate hygiene, such as vaginal douches, lubricants, or contraceptives, have been shown to kill beneficial bacteria. Besides already available probiotic creams and pills focused on improving the genital microbiome, next-generation hygiene products are certainly going to address these microbiome benefits. An example in this field is the Belgian company YUN Probiotherapy.

Microbiome-Friendly Product Claims and Certifications

Consumer goods related to the microbiome already float in the market. As usual, the marketing is running ahead of science and the customer is often helpless when choosing the correct microbiome products. For example, claims in the cosmetic industry are often based on the supplementation of pro-, pre-, and post-biotics, in most cases taken from popular knowledge about the gut microbiome which isn't much use for the skin microbiome. There are also products, which only by avoiding ingredients known to have antimicrobial activity, claim to be good for the skin's microbiome. Most skin products actually lack data behind their microbiome claims. Claims about improving the microbiome are hard to obtain and nearly impossible for healthy skin (and skin microbiome).

Clinical settings struggle with different pitfalls:

- There is not a standard healthy microbiome
- The microbiome underlies numerous influences (sex, drug use, antibiotic treatments, age, diet, lifestyle, geographical, origin, season, and even pet ownership have been shown to impact the composition of a person's skin microbiome)
- Methods used are not standardized (swab vs. strip; 16s rRNA vs. whole genome sequencing; quality of the database)

Since the ban on animal testing, in vitro methods have been validated under the guidelines of the Organisation for Economic Co-operation and Development. Given the complexity of the skin microbiome, a standardized, meaningful in vitro test is making easy for the customer to understand the results. The minimum requirement for any cosmetic should be *microbiome-friendly*—meaning it doesn't harm the skin's microbiome. MyMicrobiome is the world's first company to issue certifications for microbiome-friendly cosmetic products. The products are tested *in vitro* in a broad range of assays to determine the influence on the growth of the skin's key species. The testing includes co-cultivation as well as single-organism plate assays. If the tested product does not change the in vitro grown skin microbes, the products can be certified as microbiome-friendly.

In general, products claiming non-harmful or beneficial effects on the microbiome are gaining popularity. The food and beverage (F&B) industry is also following this trend. Besides natural pre- and pro-biotic-containing food products (kefir, kombucha, sauerkraut, kimchi etc.), a number of F&B products with pre- and pro-biotic formulations is rapidly growing. Microbiome-friendly product claims are often found in food products such as cereal bars or snacks. In the beverage sector, prebiotic juices or smoothies, and even fiber-containing carbonated (soda) drinks are available.

In summary, consumer goods related to the microbiome are already flooding the market. As usual, the marketing is running ahead of science and the customer is often helpless when choosing good microbiome products. This is why science-based product claims and learning more about microbiomes are crucial, both for consumers and producers. We hope that our book can help at least a little.

PART V

CHALLENGES OF HUMAN MICROBIOME SCIENCE

CHAPTER 18

THEIR PRESENCE INSIDE AND OUTSIDE OF US

Xenobiotics, Pollution, Antibiotics, and Microbiomes

THE earliest microbial life forms inhabited our planet around 3.42 billion years ago.[1] The first xenobiotic, or chemical compounds foreign to the living world, was synthesized 166 years back.[2] To put it simply, if the first microbes were here since year one, in comparison to it, all new chemicals synthesized by humans were around one-and-a-half seconds old. Despite that, the biochemistry of life is so fantastically efficient that within this short time interval, many microbes are already able to transform human-made chemicals into other chemicals. The predicament, however, is that we still don´t know exactly which of these chemicals are good or bad for us and to what extent.

We mentioned that microbes can transform drugs, changing their efficacy, availability, or toxicity. We also explained that microbial transformation of certain natural food components (such as betaines and choline from animal-based food), can potentially damage our health. Similar risks should be carefully evaluated for each dye, preservative, aroma, sweetener, and other xenobiotics introduced into our food.

For example, artificial sweetener cyclamate has been banned in the US, because animal studies have shown its transformation by gut microbes into carcinogenic chemical cyclohexylamine.[3]

Microbial transformations of industrial and agricultural chemicals cause various health conditions in humans and animals. A famous case was the formation of kidney stones in more than 300,000 children in

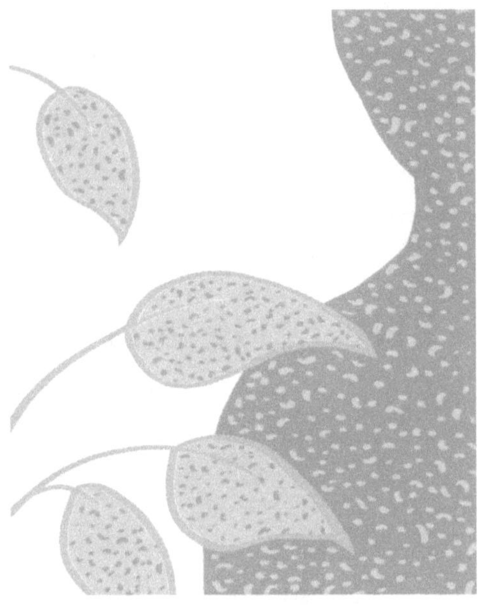

China (out of some who died), due to toxic chemical melamine, originating from plastic production, found in the baby formula.[4] Another example is nitrogen fertilizers, massively used in our agriculture since the 1950s. Excess use of nitrogen fertilizer in the soil leads to high levels of nitrates in drinking waters which, when consumed by humans and animals, are converted into carcinogenic N-nitroso compounds, most likely by our gut microbes.[5] Also, pesticides have been related to cancers, leukemia, asthma, Parkinson´s disease, cognitive disorders, and others.[6] Several studies in animals have shown microbial dysbiosis and changes in gut wall permeability as a consequence of pesticide exposures.[7] Studies in mice have shown the importance of gut microbes for elimination of heavy metals from the body.[8] Studies on microplastic accumulation in animals have shown negative effects on their microbiomes (among many other negative effects), yet unclear in humans.[9] Environmental waste pollutants, also known as endocrine disruptors (EDs), from plastics, pesticides, synthetic fertilizers, electronic waste, and food additives, are known to affect human hormones in various ways. EDs influence human metabolism (e.g. insulin resistance and diabetes), and reproductive and mental health. Mutual interaction between EDs, hormones from circulation, and metabolites produced by microbes (including hormones) have only recently gained more attention.[10] A number of studies have shown relations between air pollution, EDs, microbiome dysbiosis, and disease of respiratory and other systems and organs.[11]

In general, a decrease in microbiome diversity can have detrimental health effects. For example, antibiotic treatment can allow a single bacterial species to become dominant, as already explained in the case of *Clostridium difficile* gut infection. Unfortunately, our activities and our lifestyle are constantly decreasing the diversity of our microbiomes and our environment. Studies on indigenous human populations which have not previously been in contact with other humans, such as Hadza hunter-gatherers in Tanzania or Yanomami tribes in Amazon rain forests, have shown that their gut microbiomes have more richness and diversity, both in the number of microbial species and functions these species can perform. Interestingly, Yanomami gut microbes also have antibiotic resistance genes, suggesting either an intrinsic potential for antibiotic resistance in humans or its introduction by other indirect contacts.[12] Let's note that human microbiomes are not only also exposed to antibiotics by their use in humans but also in plants and animals. The global increase in antibiotic resistance is alarming, not only because of more danger to controlling infections, but also because of their numerous potential effects (via gut dysbiosis) on the immune system and metabolism.[13]

Biobanking

Loss of microbes over generations is resulting in permanently missing microbial species . In fact, due to the rapid changes in our diets and environments, these microbes are going extinct before we have even had the chance to study them and discover the amazing things they are capable of. To address this concern, it has been proposed that we store our microbiomes in Biobanks to preserve species before they are lost forever. Fortunately, compared to higher species of animals, bacteria are easier to preserve. For example, by suspending in a simple solution of glycerol and storing at -80 C, the majority of bacteria can remain viable for several years. Deep-freezing (cryopreservation) is also a standard for the biobanking of fungi or viruses. Another popular method for long-term biobanking of bacteria and yeast is freeze-drying (lyophilization),[14] a process in which water is removed from frozen samples, which can be afterwards stored without refrigeration. This way, it is possible to take microbes from your body and store them for thousands of years in a freezer—truly, life after death!

Microbiome in the Built Environment

Our microbiomes co-evolved with the microbes of all things around us, all our environment. Our ancestors wandered barefoot the savannah and rainforests scavenging for food, drank from rivers and ponds, and ate raw meat—even raw colon! Today, not only do we challenge microbial biodiversity through diet—eating too many processed foods filled with preservatives, and not enough fiber and fermented foods—medicines and excessive hygiene, but we've also lost touch with the outdoors. You may have heard that we now spend 90 percent of our lifespan indoors in developed countries. That's bad, and that's likely underestimated considering this figure dates to 2001[15] and we've learned to spend almost 100 percent indoors during the pandemic lockdowns since then.

The planet's fastest-growing biome is the indoor environment.

Why is that a problem? The built environment is known to be more polluted than the outdoors, including in big cities, and our walls leave little room for soil, plants, and bountiful sources of abundant microbial life. The indoors are also a major place of infectious disease transmission, as is well known for the influenza virus and *Mycobacterium tuberculosis*, and even more so in hospitals, carrier of even more dangerous pathogens, such as the Methicillin-resistant *Staphylococcus aureus* (MRSA).

Dwelling in Our Homes

Microorganisms of the human body impact the microbiome of the home, and reciprocally.

The microbiomes on the surfaces in homes vary widely depending on the occupants' microbiomes, people density and health status, presence of pets and plants, air filtration systems, humidity and temperature, and daily practices such as whether you flush the toilets with the lid open or closed. Professor and microbiome expert Jack Gilbert says we shed about 36 million microorganisms around us every hour.[16]

The Home Microbiome Project was a study of 7 families, including 3 dogs and 1 cat, and their homes. It showed that microbes shed by people impact the microbiome in the home so much you can match each person to their house based on the floor, doorknob, light switches, and keyboard samplings.[17] Three of the families moved during the study, and it took less than a day for the new house to be colonized with a similar microbial profile as the families' prior home.

"In addition to effects on health, microorganisms affect building materials and building systems, including through degradation, corrosion, and fouling as a result of biofilm formation. These effects can have economic and sustainability costs, and the varied effects and trade-offs involved will influence the assessment of potential interventions to modify indoor microbiomes."[18]

The science of building is facing important questions. For example, a way to increase occupants' health and comfort and at the same time promote exposure to a greater diversity of microorganisms is by increasing the flow of outdoor air, but it could also increase energy consumption for heating and cooling and grow exposure to allergens or other outdoor pollutants.

The construction sector is one of the major sources of greenhouse gas emissions. In consequence, one of the main goals of architectural sciences is the development of alternative materials and methods of construction, more energy-efficient, and more adaptable to environmental conditions.

Cross-pollination of life sciences, architecture, and molecular genetics brought an interesting reflection on how to mimic nature in a study from 2017,[19] interweaving biofilm communities and synthetic circuits to construct future buildings and sequester carbon dioxide in the process! The researchers' idea is to precipitate calcium carbonate by the hydration of carbon dioxide ($CO_2 + H_2O = HCO_3^- + H^+$), which provides a long-lasting cementitious material, and the researchers are already able to predict and manipulate the shape and growth of such crystals.

"The ultimate goal is to design new "intelligent," adaptable, energy-efficient materials, by integrating living cells into building and architecture," the authors say. This is the modern prolongation of Vitruvius's statement "architecture is an imitation of nature" in 27 BC.[20]

Architects are faced with new questions. Could filtration systems in the future remove pollutants and allergens while adding a healthy dose of microbes? Could building blocks be infused by bacteria and fungi to bring solidity, flexibility, isolation, aeration, serve as carbon sinks, and possibly be released little by little to increase microbial exposure?

Ioana Man is a multidisciplinary designer working at the crossroads of architecture, set design, and clinical practice who created the project "the Architectural Exposome" to change how

She encourages her contemporaries to see the building at a different spatial scale, to perceive the porosity of walls from the nano point of view, and at a different time scale, showing that the interaction with microbes participates in the structure's aging. architects think about their craft and bring them in direct contact with the microscopic world.

"The micro-world is showing clear signals of the large and slow ecological crisis we're in. We've already lost a third of microbial diversity. As we are headed towards dramatic ecological and microbial collapse, this project is to design tools that push architects to engage with ecosystems by allowing for direct interaction with the microbial."[21]

The question of improving the microbiome of the built environment is not only a matter of the builders and architects though; the occupants are also important players. Schedules of aeration, cleaning, and the choice of chemicals used in cleaning products all have an impact. You can even find probiotics for surfaces to keep your home clean and rebalance the home biome by bringing some species that could compete with unwanted molds, resistant bacteria, and allergens, like Homebiotic and BetterAir.[22] However, such consumer goods products are not required to label the microorganisms they contain, at least for now, and the companies make claims without listing scientific references, so it's still a black box.

Sound advice would be to treat your body and your home the same way you treat your gut microbiota – without antimicrobial substances, keeping in mind at each meal, each shower, each aeration, to eat, clean, and breathe also for your microbes. Jack Gilbert's mother, as he relates in the book *Dirt Is Good*,[23] says that: "A home should be clean enough to be healthy but dirty enough to be happy". Avoiding antimicrobial soaps, restoring natural habitats inside the house, nurturing plants, and getting your hands in the dirt when you can are all good habits. Washing dishes by hand also keeps more of the bacteria alive than with the dishwasher, which is a good thing.

Researchers think that the common soil bacterium *Mycobacterium vaccae* could be one of the reasons gardening is so good for mental well-being[24] so fill in these pots with your bare hands! Pets are also a good source of old friends, which could explain why children raised with dogs have 13 percent less risk of developing asthma and allergies.[25]

> "Just as bodies are not fortresses to be protected, but rather complex symbiotic systems, space is also not something to be sanitized, but rather a collection of pulsating ecosystems."
>
> —Ioana Man[26]

Life Saviors in the Hospital

The hospital's microbial environment is, more than any other built space, critical for the health of its occupants. The concentration of vulnerable people and disease make it a huge source of spreading infection. Up to 15 percent of patients develop nosocomial (hospital-acquired) infections during a stay in the healthcare facility.[27] Typical interventions to reduce the load of pathogens include increasing rates of outdoor ventilation, increasing air filtration efficiency, and employing air, water, and surface disinfection strategies. Newer approaches add the perspective of promoting indoor exposure to beneficial microorganisms.

The idea of environmental probiotics was first proposed by Hong Wang et al., in 2013 for pathogen control in plumbing systems.[28]

This is also the basis of Elisabetta Caselli's work which started in the same period. The principle of current sanitizers is to decimate bacteria. The main issue is that the surviving ones will thrive, with no competition around, and the process will select bacteria with antimicrobial substances resistance genes, leading to a higher concentration of resistant pathogens after the sanitizer is applied. Important nosocomial pathogens including MRSA, Vancomycin-resistant *Enterococci*, *Pseudomonas*, *Acinetobacter*, and viruses stay infective for days and even weeks on dry surfaces, and *C. difficile* spores can survive for months! They were found in an alarmingly high proportion of patients' rooms. Most of the chemical techniques used thus far have proven effective for the immediate abatement of the pathogen numbers, but are useless to prevent recontamination, and they come at a high environmental cost.

Elisabetta Caselli's group of research has tested the potential to switch from chemical sanitizers to probiotics based on non-pathogenic *Bacillus* spores, *B. subtilis*, *B. pumilus* and *B. megaterium* proven as safe including in vulnerable patients.[29] The scientists showed such an approach reduced recontamination by diverse pathogens by 80–90 percent compared to conventional cleansers,[30] confirmed that these spores can germinate on the treated surfaces and that they don't acquire antibiotic resistance genes, making them a safe approach to preventing the horizontal transmission of these genes to fellow microbes in the room.[31] Being infected with a MRSA leads to a 64 percent higher mortality risk compared to the non-resistant form[32] so reducing the spread of antimicrobial resistance actively saves lives.

In 2018, the team tested this probiotic approach in s hospitals in Italy and the results have been exhilarating. There was half the number of nosocomial infections in these hospitals, a decrease in pathogen load 80 percent better than the traditional disinfectant, and a decrease by 100,000 times of the antimicrobial resistance.[33] At a lesser economic cost.

At your own level, if you don't have the chance to choose which sanitizer is used in your local hospital, the simplest way to reduce the abundance of human pathogens in a hospital room is to open the windows.[34]

The World Health Organization warned in 2015 about the surge of antimicrobial resistance[35] and the advent of a new era when we would die in millions from incurable infective diseases,[36] the "post-antibiotic era". In this context, probiotics, from our gut to our hospital walls, are a huge ally.

Shaping Cities

The discovery of infectious bacteria's role in epidemics led to the creation of aqueducts, sanitation, and sewers in the 17th century.

Londoners started to build from brick rather than timber after the London Fire because it is less flammable and also because it made it difficult for rats to burrow and spread the plague.[37] In a way, microorganisms guided the cities' evolution, as they guided our gastrointestinal system's evolution.

The sewer is also taking the pulse of city inhabitants in real-time, as shown by the Underworlds studies.[38] Luigi, a robot developed by the Massachusetts Institute of Technology (MIT) spinoff, collects fecal matter in the sewer to analyze in real-time the community's collective health, monitor drug usage, predict the spread of transmissible diseases, and mitigate outbreaks. On the MIT campus, as the semester unfolds, it's possible to sense the tension from the levels of adrenaline, cortisol, and other stress biomarkers in the sewers! The Biobot even aims at identifying new coronavirus variants, to catch new threats as soon as they emerge.[39]

> "Human fecal matter is a gold mine of information. But most of it comes down to the microbiome—a collection of bacteria, virus, and fungi that live on and inside our bodies which in general, acts as a mediator of the environment and our body," explains Eric Alm, a biological engineer at the MIT who founded the Underworlds project.

We excrete information, and that wastewater could lead to "precision public health" with the right stools—uh, tools.[40]

CHAPTER 19

REGULATORY AND ETHICAL PERSPECTIVES

THE field of microbiomics is very young and its applications and products only started to flourish during the last couple of years. Therefore, it is no wonder that regulators and regulatory services accompanying these products are still in their infancy. Let's take a short look at the situation.

Authorities such as the U.S. Food and Drug Administration (FDA; for food and drug) in the U.S., or European Food Safety Authority (food) and European Medicines Agency (medical) in European Union (EU), distinguish between a food (nutritional) product and a drug. In general, regulations for food products are relatively simpler, because their target group are healthy people. In the case of therapeutics, they need to go through the phases of a clinical trial, as each drug has to be of high quality and efficacy against the particular condition, and above all, it needs to be safe.

"Probiotic" is a term which has been coined decades ago, with the goal to describe food supplements and foods containing live microbes which could replace harmful microbes in our guts. In the meantime, as the therapeutical effects of some of the probiotics became more evident, in 2016 the FDA introduced the category of Live Biotherapeutic Products or shortly LBPs.

> According to this guideline, LBP is defined as a product that:
> 1. contains live organisms, such as bacteria;
> 2. is applicable to the prevention, treatment, or cure of a disease or condition of human beings; and
> 3. is not a vaccine.[1]

However, as previously discussed in Chapter 13, the official definition of probiotics can significantly differ between different countries. In the EU, for example, a product can have the label "probiotic" only if it has a clearly demonstrated health claim, which is a long and expensive procedure, similar to drug licensing. Only a few countries such as Italy, Denmark, and Spain have approved the use of "probiotic" product labels so far. In any case and, independently of definitions and regulatory differences between countries, quicker discovery and approval of new probiotics is desperately needed. Currently, only few dozens of probiotics have been approved, which is only a tiny fraction in comparison to hundreds, if not thousands of microbes in our guts.[2]

Dozens of LBPs by different microbiome companies are currently in clinical trials. Some of them are single strains of bacteria, while others are mixtures of LBPs or so-called "microbial consortia." In 2020, SER-109, a bacterial consortium (LBP), was the first FDA-approved microbiome drug against recurring *Clostridium difficile* (rCDI), a serious gut pathogen. At the moment of writing this book, at least several other candidate LBPs are in the final, third phase of clinical trials.

The next regulatory hurdle regarding microbiome products are non-living microorganisms (postbiotics) and other microbial products such as microbial proteins, peptides, other small molecules, or metabolites. Although non-living products have a theoretical advantage over probiotics or LBPs, because they are less likely to cause inflammation (for example by reaching the bloodstream), or a disease (if they are contaminated by a living microbial pathogen), their risks and health benefits also need a clear definition by the regulatory authorities.[3] There are also dozens of candidate therapeutics in this category in clinical trials.

In Chapter 12, we described the history and applications of phage therapy. Due to historical and political circumstances, the use of phages has been widely accepted in the countries which belonged to the former Soviet Union and former "Eastern Bloc" but not in the Western countries. In 2006, a US-based company Intralytix, received the first FDA approval for use of phages for food safety. A series of other approvals in the US followed, including human therapy.[4] Unfortunately, the use of living phages in the EU is still not allowed and the companies in this area mostly rely on phage products, such as Lysins.

Technological advances in the last decades gave us opportunities to precisely engineer the genetic code of virtually any organism. Regarding microbiomes this can mean:

a) adding new functions to microbiomes by adding engineered microbes or adding new features (e.g., genes, proteins) to existing ones;

b) selectively delete microbes from a community

c) use engineered microbes for diagnostic purposes;

d) deliver vaccines, etc.

Despite the enormous possibilities, current investments in the field, and some success in animal models, there are still open regulatory and ethical issues with this approach. First, we still need to know more details about the systemic effect that a particular microbiome intervention may cause. Second, if necessary, we need to have a mechanism for the removal of engineered microbes from the organism and the environment. Also, such organisms will be considered genetically modified and may fall under different regulations in different countries.[5] Basically, there are two groups among specialists and non-specialists regarding the application of engineered microorganisms: those who like to try new options and those who consider existing natural diversity as the perfect solution. As with the application of any new technology, sufficient caution has to be taken and decisions concerning humans and the environment should be made by panels of independent experts.

EPILOGUE: WHAT THE FUTURE HOLDS

Here's the end. Let us be a little philosophical.

Microbiome research over the last two decades has led to a shift in our concept of "self."

First, our definition of self as a set of characteristics we observe is called "phenotype" and depends on how and which *genes* in our body are turned on or off. According to the estimates, the number of microbial genes, in and on our body is at least several orders of magnitude higher than the number of genes in our body's cells. Namely, if we assume there are one thousand bacterial species in the human gut (estimates are 500-1,000 species), that equals around two million genes. On the other hand, the number of genes in the human genome is around twenty thousand.[1]

Second, the main system in charge of recognizing self from non-self is our adaptive *immune system*. Throughout the book, we learned that our immune system is trained, but can be also tweaked by our microbiome.

Third, our personality and our individual perception of our self depend on our *brain*. However, our cognition is influenced by the microbiome through the microbiome *gut-brain-axis*.[2]

We can conclude that we humans are not individual entities, but rather, we live in symbiosis with a range of microscopic organisms, including bacteria, archaea, small eukaryotes, viruses, and fungi. These organisms, particularly those in our gastrointestinal tracts, act like functional organs and have a profound impact on our health. They are intricately involved in many aspects of our physiology, from influencing our mood and appetites, to how our body processes energy.

We co-evolved with these microbes over millennia. However, with recent seismic shifts in modern humanity's lifestyle and diet, the pace of change may have been too fast for our symbionts to adequately adapt. Artificial and nutritionally simple diets are selected for altered, less diverse gut bacterial communities, and as a result, an increasing number of people are living in a pre-disease state, and susceptible to chronic diseases like diabetes, obesity, inflammatory bowel disease, and others. Interventions and treatments will be required to modulate our gut health in the face of our changing habits.

Except for philosophical challenges, there are still many practical, scientific questions about microbiomes that are waiting to be answered. For example, by which environmental signals, which microbial genes turn on or off? Which molecular signals do they provide to the body cells and organs and vice versa, how do the other organs and organic systems exactly "talk" to the microbiomes? How do the individual genetic differences and the differences in the way we develop in our mother's womb and the way we are delivered and raised in the first days and months, influence the structures of an individual's microbiomes? Future studies will need to account for inter-individual variation in microbial communities. The future will be personalized—effective strategies for nutrition, supplementation, and disease treatment will all have to consider the condition and composition of our individual microbiomes.

Technology is moving forward at a stunning pace. New sequencing devices size of our palms are available, with the ever-higher length and precision of reading and lower prices. "Omics" technologies are enabling us to reassemble thousands of genes and analyze RNA, proteins, and metabolites. However, our techniques to precisely isolate, identify, and culture the remaining 99 percent of microbial "black matter" are not there yet. Computer processors are becoming more powerful, new algorithms for extracting meaningful information from huge amounts of data and artificial intelligence are a thriving field of research. Still, there is a lot of work to be done: standardization of workflows and databases and integration of "omics" technologies are far from perfect. New banks for storing single microbes, microbial consortia, small molecules, and other samples for future therapies and research are urgently needed. Standardization is required for microbiome research studies as well as for clinical ones. The regulatory framework regarding manufacturing, labeling, safety, stability, and other features needed for introducing new microbiome therapeutics such as live bacterial products, phages, and others, should be accelerated and unified between different geographies.

As we learn more about our microbes, we will develop strategies to harness the microbial world to our advantage. The direction of these strategies will be accelerated by developments in microbiome research, which is perhaps the most exciting area in biology right now. We can expect greater integration of different fields such as microbiology, immunology, biochemistry, nutrition, physiology, genetics, statistics, and bioinformatics. Reduction in sequencing costs will facilitate more studies with more detail and greater depth, as we will be able to include more samples across different time points. To complement these studies, mechanistic analyses and bench-work science will help deduce causality from association, which is a limitation of much of our current research.

Last but not least, more public awareness about achievements and potential in microbiome science is needed and, as already stated, this was the motivation behind writing this book. Although the microbiome "hype" is gaining momentum worldwide, any kind of pseudo-science, charlatanism, and unadvised or unsafe application of microbiomes must be avoided. In this sense regular education of the broad public, doctors, nutritionists, and other specialists is essential.

By spreading awareness about the importance of a microbiome-conscious living environment, nutrition, active lifestyle, and therapy, we hope to move one step closer to improving our health, our quality of life, and our longevity!

NOTES AND REFERENCES

Chapter 1

1. "Human Genome Project," https://www.genome.gov/human-genome-project
2. Jeremy Preston, Asley VanZeeland, and Daniel A. Peiffer, "Innovation at Illumina: The Road to the $600 Human Genome," *Nature Portfolio*, https://www.nature.com/articles/d42473-021-00030-9
3. Peter J. Turnbaugh et al., "The Human Microbiome Project," *Nature* 449, no. 7164 (2007): 804–10.
4. Manon Boxberger et al., "Challenges in Exploring and Manipulating the Human Skin Microbiome," *Microbiome* 9, no. 1 (2021): 125.
5. Sara Saheb Kashaf et al., "Integrating Cultivation and Metagenomics for a Multi-kingdom View of Skin Microbiome Diversity and Functions," *Nature Microbiology* 7, no. 1 (2022): 169–79.
6. Rob Knight and Brendan Buhler, *Follow Your Gut: The Enormous Impact of Tiny Microbes* (London: Simon & Schuster, 2015).
7. Vinod K. Gupta, Sandip Paul, and Chitra Dutta, "Geography, Ethnicity or Subsistence-Specific Variations in Human Microbiome Composition and Diversity," *Frontiers in Microbiology* 8 (2017): 1162.
8. Priya Nimish Deo and Revati Deshmukh, "Oral Microbiome: Unveiling the Fundamentals," *Journal of Oral and Maxillofacial Pathology* 23, no. 1 (2019): 122–8.
9. David N. O'Dwyer, Robert P. Dickson, and Bethany B. Moore, "The Lung Microbiome, Immunity, and the Pathogenesis of Chronic Lung Disease," *Journal of Immunology* 196, no. 12 (2016): 4839–47.
10. D. Scott et al., "The Life and Death of Helicobacter pylori," *Gut* 43 Suppl. 1 (1998): S56–60.
11. Jing Yang et al., "Species-Level Analysis of Human Gut Microbiota with Metataxonomics," *Frontiers in Microbiology* 11 (2020): 2029; Mirjana Rajilić-Stojanović and Willem M. de Vos, "The First 1000 Cultured Species of the Human Gastrointestinal Microbiota," *FEMS Microbiology Reviews* 38, no. 5 (2014): 996–1047.

12. Elizabeth Thursby and Nathalie Juge, "Introduction to the Human Gut Microbiota," *Biochemical Journal* 474, no. 11 (2017): 1823–36.

13. Samantha A. Whiteside et al., "The Microbiome of the Urinary Tract—a Role Beyond Infection," *Nature Reviews. Urology* 12, no. 2 (2015): 81–90.

14. Harris Onywera et al., "The Penile Microbiota in Uncircumcised and Circumcised Men: Relationships with HIV and Human Papillomavirus Infections and Cervicovaginal Microbiota," *Frontiers in Medicine* 7 (2020): 383.

15. Viqar Sayeed Saraf et al., "Vaginal Microbiome: Normalcy vs Dysbiosis," *Archives of Microbiology* 203, no. 7 (2021): 3793–802; Sam Schoenmakers and Joop Laven, "The Vaginal Microbiome as a Tool to Predict IVF Success," *Current Opinion in Obstetrics and Gynecology* 32, no. 3 (2020): 169–78.

16. Schoenmakers, S. & Laven, J. The vaginal microbiome as a tool to predict IVF success. Current Opinion in Obstetrics & Gynecology 32, 169–178 (2020).

Chapter 2

1. Samuel A. Smits et al., "Seasonal Cycling in the Gut Microbiome of the Hadza Hunter-Gatherers of Tanzania," *Science* (New York, NY) 357, no. 6353 (2017): 802–6.

2. Kazuhiro Ogai et al., "A Comparison of Techniques for Collecting Skin Microbiome Samples: Swabbing Versus Tape-Stripping," *Frontiers in Microbiology* 9 (2018): 2362.

3. Egija Zaura et al., "Optimizing the Quality of Clinical Studies on Oral Microbiome: A Practical Guide for Planning, Performing, and Reporting," *Periodontology 2000* 85, no. 1 (2021): 210–36.

4. "The Gut Microbiome," https://www.pelican-health.com/

5. Q. Tang et al., "Current Sampling Methods for Gut Microbiota: A Call for More Precise Devices," *Frontiers in Cellular and Infection Microbiology* 10 (2020): 151.

6. Seppo Virtanen et al., "Comparative Analysis of Vaginal Microbiota Sampling Using 16S RRNA Gene Analysis," *PLoS One* 12, no. 7 (2017): e0181477.

7. Angie Mordant and Manuel Kleiner, "Evaluation of Sample Preservation and Storage Methods for Metaproteomics Analysis of Intestinal Microbiomes," *Microbiology Spectrum* 9, no. 3 (2021): e0187721.

8. E. M. Terveer et al., "How to: Establish and Run a Stool Bank," *Clinical Microbiology and Infection* 23, no. 12 (2017): 924–30; Simon Mark Dahl Baunwall et al., "The Use of Faecal Microbiota Transplantation (FMT) in Europe: A Europe-Wide Survey," *Lancet Regional Health. Europe* 9 (2021): 100181.

Chapter 3

1. M. Bonnet et al., "Bacterial Culture Through Selective and Non-selective Conditions: the Evolution of Culture Media in Clinical Microbiology," *New Microbes and New Infections* 34 (2020).

2. T. Sandle, "History and Development of Microbiological Culture Media," *The Journal. (Institute of Science and Technology)* (2010): 10–4.

3. Muriel C. F. van Teeseling, and Christian Jogler, "Cultivation of Elusive Microbes Unearthed Exciting Biology," *Nature Communications* 12, no. 1 (2021): 75.

4. M. Minekus, "The TNO Gastro-Intestinal Model (TIM)," in *The Impact of Food Bioactives on Health: In Vitro and Ex Vivo Models*, ed. K. Verhoeckx et al (Cham [CH]: Springer 2015); Rocío García-Villalba et al., "Gastrointestinal Simulation Model TWIN-SHIME Shows Differences Between Human Urolithin-Metabotypes in Gut Microbiota Composition, Pomegranate Polyphenol Metabolism, and Transport Along the Intestinal Tract," *Journal of Agricultural and Food Chemistry* 65, no. 27 (2017): 5480–93.

5. Shafaque Rahman et al., "The Progress of Intestinal Epithelial Models from Cell Lines to Gut-On-Chip," *International Journal of Molecular Sciences* 22, no. 24 (2021): 13472.

6. Ibid.

7. Elizabeth A. Kennedy, Katherine Y. King, and Megan T. Baldridge, "Mouse Microbiota Models: Comparing Germ-Free Mice and Antibiotics Treatment as Tools for Modifying Gut Bacteria," *Frontiers in Physiology* 9 (2018): 1534.

8. Angela E. Douglas, "Simple Animal Models for Microbiome Research," *Nature Reviews. Microbiology* 17, no. 12 (2019): 764–75.

Chapter 4

1. Louise Walsh, "Journeys of Discovery," https://www.cam.ac.uk/stories/journeys ofdiscovery-rapidgenomesequencing

2. Shawn E. Levy and Braden E. Boone, "Next-Generation Sequencing Strategies," *Cold Spring Harbor Perspectives in Medicine* 9, no. 7 (2019): a025791; Louise Walsh, "Journeys of Discovery," https://www.cam.ac.uk/stories/journeys ofdiscovery-rapidgenomesequencing

3. Jonathan M. Rothberg et al., "An Integrated Semiconductor Device Enabling Non-optical Genome Sequencing," *Nature* 475, no. 7356 (2011): 348–52.

4. Rupesh Kanchi Ravi, Kendra Walton, and Mahdieh Khosroheidari, "MiSeq: A Next Generation Sequencing Platform for Genomic Analysis," *Methods in Molecular Biology* 1706 (2018): 223–32.

5. Malla, M. A., Dubey, A., Kumar, A., Yadav, S., Hashem, A., and Abd_Allah, E. F., "Exploring the Human Microbiome: The Potential Future Role of Next-Generation Sequencing in Disease Diagnosis and Treatment," *Frontiers in Immunology* 9, 2868 (2019).

6. Jeanette L. Gehrig, Daniel M. Portik, Mark D. Driscoll, Eric Jackson, Shreyasee Chakraborty, Dawn Gratalo, Meredith Ashby, and Ricardo Valladares, "Finding the right fit: A comprehensive evaluation of short-read and long-read

sequencing approaches to maximize the utility of clinical microbiome data," *bioRxiv* (2021).08.31.458285.

7. Neelja Singhal et al., "MALDI-TOF Mass Spectrometry: an Emerging Technology for Microbial Identification and Diagnosis," *Frontiers in Microbiology* 6 (2015): 791; Suresh Kumar Kailasa et al., "Progress of Electrospray Ionization and Rapid Evaporative Ionization Mass Spectrometric Techniques for the Broad-Range Identification of Microorganisms," *Analyst* 144, no. 4 (2019): 1073–103..

8. Saleh Alseekh et al., "Mass Spectrometry-Based Metabolomics: A Guide for Annotation, Quantification and Best Reporting Practices," *Nature Methods* 18, no. 7 (2021): 747–56.

9. Jean-Christophe Lagier et al., "Culturing the Human Microbiota and Culturomics," *Nature Reviews. Microbiology* 16 (2018): 540–50.

Chapter 5

1. Ana Elena Pérez-Cobas, Laura Gomez-Valero, and Carmen Buchrieser, "Metagenomic Approaches in Microbial Ecology: an Update on Whole-Genome and Marker Gene Sequencing Analyses," *Microbial Genomics* 6, no. 8 (2020).

2. Julia K. Goodrich et al., "Conducting a Microbiome Study," *Cell* 158, no. 2 (2014): 250–62.

3. Rob Knight et al., "Best Practices for Analysing Microbiomes," *Nature Reviews. Microbiology* 16, no. 7 (2018): 410–22.

4. Jessica Gambardella, Vanessa Castellanos, and Gaetano Santulli, "Standardizing Translational Microbiome Studies and Metagenomic Analyses," *Cardiovascular Research* 117, no. 3 (2021): 640–2.

5. Duo Jiang et al, "Microbiome Multi-omics Network Analysis: Statistical Considerations, Limitations, and Opportunities," *Frontiers in Genetics* 10 (2019): 995; Laura E. McCoubrey et al., "Harnessing Machine Learning for Development of Microbiome Therapeutics," *Gut Microbes* 13, no. 1 (2021): 1–20; Junghyun Namkung, "Machine Learning Methods for Microbiome Studies," *Journal of Microbiology* 58, no. 3 (2020): 206–16.

Chapter 6

1. Fredrik Bäckhed et al., "Defining a Healthy Human Gut Microbiome: Current Concepts, Future Directions, and Clinical Applications," *Cell Host and Microbe* 12, no. 5 (2012): 611–22.

2. Albert Palleja et al., "Recovery of Gut Microbiota of Healthy Adults Following Antibiotic Exposure," *Nature Microbiology* 3, no. 11 (2018): 1255–65.

3. Jeremiah J. Faith et al., "The Long-Term Stability of the Human Gut Microbiota," *Science* 341, no. 6141 (2013): 1237439.

4. Dirk Gevers et al., "The Human Microbiome Project: a Community Resource for the Healthy Human Microbiome," *PLOS Biology* 10, no. 8 (2012): e1001377.

5. Gevers et al., "The Human Microbiome Project," e1001377; Julia K. Goodrich et al., "Human Genetics Shape the Gut Microbiome," *Cell* 159, no. 4 (2014): 789–99; Gwen Falony et al., "Population-Level Analysis of Gut Microbiome Variation," *Science* 352, no. 6285 (2016): 560–4; Andrew W. Brooks et al., "Gut Microbiota Diversity Across Ethnicities in the United States," *PLOS Biology* 16, no. 12 (2018): e2006842; Daniel McDonald et al., "American Gut: an Open Platform for Citizen Science Microbiome Research," *mSystems* 3, no. 3 (2018); Daphna Rothschild et al., "Environment Dominates over Host Genetics in Shaping Human Gut Microbiota," *Nature* 555, no. 7695 (2018): 210–5; Robert C. Kaplan et al., "Gut Microbiome Composition in the Hispanic Community Health Study/Study of Latinos Is Shaped by Geographic Relocation, Environmental Factors, and Obesity," *Genome Biology* 20, no. 1 (2019): 219.

6. Joseph M. Pickard et al., "Gut Microbiota: Role in Pathogen Colonization, Immune Responses, and Inflammatory Disease," *Immunological Reviews* 279, no. 1 (2017): 70–89.

7. Ohad Manor et al., "Health and Disease Markers Correlate with Gut Microbiome Composition Across Thousands of People," *Nature Communications* 11, no. 1 (2020): 5206.

8. Yue Xiao et al., "Human Gut-Derived *B. longum* Subsp. *longum* strains protect against aging in a D-galactose-induced aging mouse model," *Microbiome* 9, no. 1 (2021).

9. Tyrrell Conway and Paul S. Cohen, "Commensal and Pathogenic Escherichia coli Metabolism in the Gut," *Microbiology Spectrum* 3, no. 3 (2015).

10. Jose U. Scher et al., "Expansion of Intestinal Prevotella copri Correlates with Enhanced Susceptibility to Arthritis," *eLife* 2 (2013): e01202; Adrian Tett et al., "The Prevotella copri Complex Comprises Four Distinct Clades Underrepresented in Westernized Populations," *Cell Host and Microbe* 26, no. 5 (2019): 666–679.e7.

11. Cormac Brian Fitzgerald et al., "Comparative Analysis of Faecalibacterium prausnitzii Genomes Shows a High Level of Genome Plasticity and Warrants Separation into New Species-Level Taxa," *BMC Genomics* 19, no. 1 (2018): 931.

12. Nicolai Karcher et al., "Analysis of 1321 Eubacterium rectale Genomes from Metagenomes Uncovers Complex Phylogeographic Population Structure and Subspecies Functional Adaptations," *Genome Biology* 21, no. 1 (2020): 138; Yijia Wang et al., "Eubacterium rectale Contributes to Colorectal Cancer Initiation via Promoting Colitis," *Gut Pathogens* 13, no. 1 (2021): 2.

13. Yan Shao et al., "Stunted Microbiota and Opportunistic Pathogen Colonization in Caesarean-Section Birth," *Nature* 574, no. 7776 (2019): 117–21.

14. Victoria Ronan, Rummanu Yeasin, and Erika C. Claud, "Childhood Development and the Microbiome: The Intestinal Microbiota in Maintenance of Health and

Development of Disease During Childhood Development," *Gastroenterology* 160, no. 2 (2021): 495–506.

15. Kirsty Le Doare et al., "Mother's Milk: A Purposeful Contribution to the Development of the Infant Microbiota and Immunity," *Frontiers in Immunology* 9 (2018): 361; Lorena Ruiz, Cristina García-Carral, and Juan Miguel Rodriguez, "Unfolding the Human Milk Microbiome Landscape in the Omicsera," *Frontiers in Microbiology* 10 (2019): 1378.

16. David R. Hill, Jo May Chow, and Rachael H. Buck, "Multifunctional Benefits of Prevalent HMOs: Implications for Infant Health," *Nutrients* 13, no. 10 (2021): 3364.

17. Suzanne Havstad et al., "Effect of Prenatal Indoor Pet Exposure on the Trajectory of Total IgE Levels in Early Childhood," *Journal of Allergy and Clinical Immunology* 128, no. 4 (2011): 880–885.e4; Martin Depner et al., "Maturation of the Gut Microbiome During the First Year of Life Contributes to the Protective Farm Effect on Childhood Asthma," *Nature Medicine* 26, no. 11 (2020): 1766–75.

18. Derrick M. Chu et al., "Maturation of the Infant Microbiome Community Structure and Function Across Multiple Body Sites and in Relation to Mode of Delivery," *Nature Medicine* 23, no. 3 (2017): 314–26.

19. Rothschild et al., "Environment Dominates over Host Genetics in Shaping Human Gut Microbiota," 210–5.

20. Jiyoung Ahn and Richard B. Hayes, "Environmental Influences on the Human Microbiome and Implications for Noncommunicable Disease," *Annual Review of Public Health* 42 (2021): 277–92.

21. S. L. Schnorr et al., "Gut Microbiome of the Hadza Hunter-Gatherers," *Nature Communications* 51, no. 5 (2014): 1–12; Maria G. Dominguez Bello et al., "Preserving Microbial Diversity," *Science* 362, no. 6410 (2018): 33–4; S. Das et al., 'The Gut Microbiome in Western and Indigenous Cultures,' *Preprints* (2021): 2021040175.

22. Gabriela K. Fragiadakis et al., "Links Between Environment, Diet, and the Hunter-Gatherer Microbiome," *Gut Microbes* 10, no. 2 (2019): 216–27.

23. Niv Zmora, Jotham Suez, and Eran Elinav, "You Are What You Eat: Diet, Health and the Gut Microbiota," *Nature Reviews. Gastroenterology and Hepatology* 16, no. 16 (2018): 35–56.

24. Sahar El Aidy et al., "The Gut Microbiota and Mucosal Homeostasis: Colonized at Birth or at Adulthood, Does It Matter?" *Gut Microbes* 4, no. 2 (2013): 118–24.

25. Mariana X. Byndloss, Sandy R. Pernitzsch, and Andreas J. Bäumler, "Healthy Hosts Rule Within: Ecological Forces Shaping the Gut Microbiota," *Mucosal Immunology* 11, no. 5 (2018): 1299–305.

26. Valerio Iebba et al., "Eubiosis and Dysbiosis: the Two Sides of the Microbiota," *New Microbiologica* 39, no. 1 (2016): 1–12; Gabriele Berg et al., "Microbiome Definition Re-visited: Old Concepts and New Challenges," *Microbiome* 8, no.

1 (2020): 103; Harald Brüssow, "Problems with the Concept of Gut Microbiota Dysbiosis," *Microbial Biotechnology* 13, no. 2 (2020): 423–34.

27. Iebba et al., "Eubiosis and Dysbiosis: the Two Sides of the Microbiota," 1–12.

28. https://microbiomeconservancy.org/

Chapter 7

1. Wei-Ting Chen et al., "Spatial Transcriptomics and In Situ Sequencing to Study Alzheimer's Disease," *Cell* 182, no. 4 (2020): 976–991.e19.

2. Edda Russo et al. (2022), "SARS-CoV-2 and Microbiota," in ed. Gaurav Gupta, Brain G. Oliver, Kamal Dua, Alisha Singh, and Ronan MacLoughlin, *Microbiome in Inflammatory Lung Diseases*, Singapore: Springer.

3. Thomas Gensollen et al., "How Colonization by Microbiota in Early Life Shapes the Immune System," *Science* 352, no. 6285 (2016): 539–44.

4. Maka Mshvildadze, Josef Neu, and Volker Mai, "Intestinal Microbiota Development in the Premature Neonate: Establishment of a Lasting Commensal Relationship?" *Nutrition Reviews* 66, no. 11 (2008): 658–63.

5. Astrid Konrad et al., "Tight Mucosal Compartmentation of the Murine Immune Response to Antigens of the Enteric Microbiota," *Gastroenterology* 130, no. 7 (2006): 2050–9; Yasmine Belkaid and Shruti Naik, "Compartmentalized and Systemic Control of Tissue Immunity by Commensals," *Nature Immunology* 14, no. 7 (2013): 646–53.

6. Yasmine Belkaid and Shruti Naik, "Compartmentalized and Systemic Control of Tissue Immunity by Commensals," *Nature Immunology* 14, no. 7 (2013): 646–53.

7. Charles L. Bevins and Nita H. Salzman, "Paneth Cells, Antimicrobial Peptides and Maintenance of Intestinal Homeostasis," *Nature Reviews. Microbiology* 9, no. 5 (2011): 356–68.

8. Judith Wendler et al., "Proteolytic Degradation of Reduced Human Beta Defensin 1 Generates a Novel Antibiotic Octapeptide," *Scientific Reports* 9, no. 1 (2019): 3640.

9. Daniel A. Peterson et al., "IgA Response to Symbiotic Bacteria as a Mediator of Gut Homeostasis," *Cell Host and Microbe* 2, no. 5 (2007): 328–39.

10. Duncan B. Sutherland, Keiichiro Suzuki, and Sidonia Fagarasan, "Fostering of Advanced Mutualism with Gut Microbiota by Immunoglobulin A," *Immunological Reviews* 270, no. 1 (2016): 20–31.

11. Silvia Bellando-Randone et al., "Exploring the Oral Microbiome in Rheumatic Diseases, State of Art and Future Prospective in Personalized Medicine with an AI Approach," *Journal of Personalized Medicine* 11, no. 7 (2021): 625.

12. Deshire Alpizar-Rodriguez et al., "*Prevotella copri* in Individuals At Risk for Rheumatoid Arthritis," *Annals of the Rheumatic Diseases* 78, no. 5 (2019): 590–3

13. Xuan Zhang et al., "The Oral and Gut Microbiomes Are Perturbed in Rheumatoid Arthritis and Partly Normalized After Treatment," *Nature Medicine* 21, no. 8 (2015): 895–905.

14. Sabrina G. de Aquino et al., "Periodontal Pathogens Directly Promote Autoimmune Experimental Arthritis by Inducing a TLR2- and IL-1-Driven Th17 Response," *Journal of Immunology* 192, no. 9 (2014): 4103–11.

15. Addie Dissick et al., "Association of Periodontitis with Rheumatoid Arthritis: A Pilot Study," *Journal of Periodontology* 81, no. 2 (2010): 223–30.

16. Katarzyna Białowąs et al., "Periodontal Disease and Influence of Periodontal Treatment on Disease Activity in Patients with Rheumatoid Arthritis and Spondyloarthritis," *Rheumatology International* 40, no. 3 (2020): 455–63.

17. Gökhan S. Hotamisligil, "Inflammation, Metaflammation and Immunometabolic Disorders," *Nature* 542, no. 7640 (2017): 177–85.

18. Herbert Tilg et al., "The Intestinal Microbiota Fuelling Metabolic Inflammation," *Nature Reviews. Immunology* 20, no. 1 (2020): 40–54.

19. Robert A. Koeth et al., "l-Carnitine in Omnivorous Diets Induces an Atherogenic Gut Microbial Pathway in Humans," *Journal of Clinical Investigation* 129, no. 1 (2019): 373–87.

20. Kenneth Dickstein et al., "ESC Guidelines for the Diagnosis and Treatment of Acute and Chronic Heart Failure 2008: the Task Force for the Diagnosis and Treatment of Acute and Chronic Heart Failure 2008 of the European Society of Cardiology. Developed in Collaboration with the Heart Failure Association of the ESC (HFA) and Endorsed by the European Society of Intensive Care Medicine (ESICM)," *European Journal of Heart Failure* 10, no. 10 (2008): 933–89.

21. Kamyar Kalantar-Zadeh et al., "Nutritional and Anti-Inflammatory Interventions in Chronic Heart Failure," *American Journal of Cardiology* 101, no. 11A (2008): 89E–103E.

22. https://www.healthydietforhealthylife.eu/index.php/projects/research-area-supported-project/report/341; http://ambrosia-euproject.com/

23. Serban Gologan et al., "Inflammatory Gene Expression Profiles in Crohn's Disease and Ulcerative Colitis: a Comparative Analysis Using a Reverse Transcriptase Multiplex Ligation-Dependent Probe Amplification Protocol," *Journal of Crohn's and Colitis* 7, no. 8 (2013): 622–30.

24. Heitor S. P. de Souza and Claudio Fiocchi, "Immunopathogenesis of IBD: Current State of the Art," *Nature Reviews. Gastroenterology and Hepatology* 13, no. 1 (2016): 13–27.

25. Floris Imhann et al., "Interplay of Host Genetics and Gut Microbiota Underlying the Onset and Clinical Presentation of Inflammatory Bowel Disease," *Gut* 67, no. 1 (2018): 108–19.

26. Edda Russo et al., "Immunomodulating Activity and Therapeutic Effects of Short Chain Fatty Acids and Tryptophan Post-biotics in Inflammatory Bowel Disease," *Frontiers in Immunology* 10 (2019): 2754.

27. Dianne H. Dapito et al., "Promotion of Hepatocellular Carcinoma by the Intestinal Microbiota and TLR4," *Cancer Cell* 21, no. 4 (2012): 504–16.

28. Yu Zhan et al., "Gut Microbiota Protects Against Gastrointestinal Tumorigenesis Caused by Epithelial Injury," *Cancer Research* 73, no. 24 (2013): 7199–210.

29. M. Fukata and M. T. Abreu, "Role of Toll-Like Receptors in Gastrointestinal Malignancies," *Oncogene* 27, no. 2 (2008): 234–43.

30. Alberto Mantovani et al., "Cancer-Related Inflammation," *Nature* 454, no. 7203 (2008): 436–44.

31. As reviewed in Antonio Russo et al., "Multidimensional Assessment of the Effects of Erenumab in Chronic Migraine Patients with Previous Unsuccessful Preventive Treatments: a Comprehensive Real-World Experience," *Journal of Headache and Pain* 21, no. 1 (2020): 69.

32. Yun Kit Yeoh et al., "Gut Microbiota Composition Reflects Disease Severity and Dysfunctional Immune Responses in Patients with COVID-19," *Gut* 70, no. 4 (2021): 698–706.

33. Caiyun Zhang et al., "The Psychological Impact of the COVID-19 Pandemic on Teenagers in China," *Journal of Adolescent Health* (Official Publication of the Society for Adolescent Medicine) 67, no. 6 (2020): 747–55.

Chapter 8

1. James D. Schiffbauer et al., "Discovery of Bilaterian-Type Through-Guts in Cloudinomorphs from the Terminal Ediacaran Period," *Nature Communications* 11, no. 1 (2020): 205.

2. John F. Cryan et al., "The Microbiota-Gut-Brain Axis," *Physiological Reviews* 99, no. 4 (2019): 1877–2013.

3. Jessica M. Yano et al., "Indigenous Bacteria from the Gut Microbiota Regulate Host Serotonin Biosynthesis," *Cell* 161, no. 2 (2015): 264–76; Miles Berger, John A. Gray, and Bryan L. Roth, "The Expanded Biology of Serotonin," *Annual Review of Medicine* 60 (2009): 355–66.

4. Timothy G. Dinan and John F. Cryan, "The Microbiome-Gut-Brain Axis in Health and Disease," *Gastroenterology Clinics of North America* 46, no. 1 (2017): 77–89; Jason M. Peirce, and Karina Alviña, "The Role of Inflammation and the Gut Microbiome in Depression and Anxiety," *Journal of Neuroscience Research* 97, no. 10 (2019): 1223–41.

5. Leon M. T. Dicks, Diron Hurn, and Demi Hermanus, "Gut Bacteria and Neuropsychiatric Disorders," *Microorganisms* 9, no. 12 (2021): 2583.

6. Hallie R. Wachsmuth, Savanna N. Weninger, and Frank A. Duca, "Role of the Gut–Brain Axis in Energy and Glucose Metabolism," *Experimental and Molecular Medicine* 54, no. 4 (2022): 377–92.

7. The GBD 2015 Obesity Collaborators et al., "Health Effects of Overweight and Obesity in 195 Countries Over 25 Years," *New England Journal of Medicine* 377, no. 1 (2017): 13–27.

8. Peter J. Turnbaugh et al., "Diet-Induced Obesity Is Linked to Marked but Reversible Alterations in the Mouse Distal Gut Microbiome," *Cell Host and Microbe* 3, no. 4 (2008): 213–23.

9. Aline Corado Gomes, Christian Hoffmann, and João Felipe Mota, "The Human Gut Microbiota: Metabolism and Perspective in Obesity," *Gut Microbes* 9, no. 4 (2018): 308–25.

10. Arpita Arora et al., "Unravelling the Involvement of Gut Microbiota in Type 2 Diabetes Mellitus," *Life Sciences* 273 (2021): 119311.

11. Yong Fan, and Oluf Pedersen, "Gut Microbiota in Human Metabolic Health and Disease," *Nature Reviews. Microbiology* 19, no. 1 (2021): 55–71.

12. C. McDowell, and M. Haseeb. *Inflammatory Bowel Diseases (IBD)* (2017).

13. Joana Torres et al., "Crohn's Disease," *Lancet* 389, no. 10080 (2017): 1741–55

14. Kelvin T. Thia et al., "Risk Factors Associated with Progression to Intestinal Complications of Crohn's Disease in a Population-Based Cohort," *Gastroenterology* 139, no. 4 (2010): 1147–55.

15. Xochitl C. Morgan et al., "Dysfunction of the Intestinal Microbiome in Inflammatory Bowel Disease and Treatment," *Genome Biology* 13, no. 9 (2012): R79.

16. Jason M. Norman et al., "Disease-Specific Alterations in the Enteric Virome in Inflammatory Bowel Disease," *Cell* 160, no. 3 (2015): 447–60.

17. Victoria Pascal et al., "A Microbial Signature for Crohn's Disease," *Gut* 66, no. 5 (2017): 813–22.

18. Mohammad Tauqeer Alam et al., "Microbial Imbalance in Inflammatory Bowel Disease Patients at Different Taxonomic Levels," *Gut Pathogens* 12, no. 1 (2020): 1; P. Seksik et al., "Alterations of the Dominant Faecal Bacterial Groups in Patients with Crohn's Disease of the Colon," *Gut* 52, no. 2 (2003): 237–42.

19. Uri Gophna et al., "Differences Between Tissue-Associated Intestinal Microfloras of Patients with Crohn's Disease and Ulcerative Colitis," *Journal of Clinical Microbiology* 44, no. 11 (2006): 4136–41; Harry Sokol et al., "Faecalibacterium prausnitzii Is an Anti-Inflammatory Commensal Bacterium Identified by Gut Microbiota Analysis of Crohn Disease Patients," *Proceedings of the National Academy of Sciences of the United States of America* 105, no. 43 (2008): 16731–6.

20. Kathleen Machiels et al., "A Decrease of the Butyrate-Producing Species Roseburia hominis and Faecalibacterium prausnitzii Defines Dysbiosis in Patients with Ulcerative Colitis," *Gut* 63, no. 8 (2014): 1275–83; Dirk Gevers et al., "The Treatment-Naive Microbiome in New-Onset Crohn's Disease," *Cell Host and Microbe* 15, no. 3 (2014): 382–92; Nadine Fornelos et al., "Growth Effects of N-acylethanolamines on Gut Bacteria Reflect Altered Bacterial Abundances

in Inflammatory Bowel Disease," *Nature Microbiology* 5, no. 3 (2020): 486–97; Guangcai Liang, "Altered Gut Bacterial and Metabolic Signatures and Their Interaction in Inflammatory Bowel Disease," *Synthetic and Systems Biotechnology* 6, no. 4 (2021): 377–83.

21. Melanie Schirmer et al., "Dynamics of Metatranscription in the Inflammatory Bowel Disease Gut Microbiome," *Nature Microbiology* 3, no. 3 (2018): 337–46; Julian R. Marchesi et al., "Rapid and Noninvasive Metabonomic Characterization of Inflammatory Bowel Disease," *Journal of Proteome Research* 6, no. 2 (2007): 546–51; Feng Yang et al. *Journal of Separation Science* 32, no. 17 (2009): 2974–8.

22. Morgan et al., "Dysfunction of the Intestinal Microbiome in Inflammatory Bowel Disease and Treatment," R79; Feng Yang et al. *Journal of Separation Science* 32, no. 17 (2009): 2974–8.

23. Shenghua Gu et al., "Bacterial Community Mapping of the Mouse Gastrointestinal Tract," *PLoS One* 8, no. 10 (2013): e74957; Daniel A. Peterson et al., "Metagenomic Approaches for Defining the Pathogenesis of Inflammatory Bowel Diseases," *Cell Host and Microbe* 3, no. 6 (2008): 417–27.

24. Iliyan D. Iliev et al., "Interactions Between Commensal Fungi and the C-Type Lectin Receptor Dectin-1 Influence Colitis," *Science* 336, no. 6086 (2012): 1314–7.

25. Qiurong Li et al., "Dysbiosis of Gut Fungal Microbiota Is Associated with Mucosal Inflammation in Crohn's Disease," *Journal of Clinical Gastroenterology* 48, no. 6 (2014): 513–23; Christel Chehoud et al., "Fungal Signature in the Gut Microbiota of Pediatric Patients with Inflammatory Bowel Disease," *Inflammatory Bowel Diseases* 21, no. 8 (2015): 1948–56; J. D. Lewis et al., "Inflammation, Antibiotics, and Diet as Environmental Stressors of the Gut Microbiome in Pediatric Crohn's Disease," *Cell Host and Microbe* 18, no. 4 (2015): 489–500.

26. F. C. Lessa et al., "Burden of Clostridium difficile Infection in the United States," *New England Journal of Medicine* 372, no. 9 (2015): 825–34.

27. Ciarán P. Kelly, and J. Thomas LaMont, "Clostridium difficile — More Difficult than Ever," *New England Journal of Medicine* 359, no. 18 (2008): 1932–40; Michael C. Abt, Peter T. McKenney, and Eric G. Pamer, "Clostridium difficile Colitis: Pathogenesis and Host Defence," *Nature Reviews. Microbiology* 14, no. 10 (2016): 609–20; Robert P. Smith et al., "Gut Microbiome Diversity Is Associated with Sleep Physiology in Humans," *PloS One* 14, no. 10 (2019): e0222394.

28. Francesco Valitutti, Salvatore Cucchiara, and Alessio Fasano, "Celiac Disease and the Microbiome," *Nutrients* 11, no. 10 (2019): 2403.

Chapter 9

1. Britta De Pessemier et al., "Gut-Skin Axis: Current Knowledge of the Interrelationship Between Microbial Dysbiosis and Skin Conditions," *Microorganisms* 9, no. 2 (2021): 353.

2. Breck Thrash et al., "Cutaneous manifestations of gastrointestinal disease (Part II)," *Journal of the American Academy of Dermatology,* 68, no. 2 (2013): P211. E1-211.E33.

3. Pessemier et al., "Gut-Skin Axis: Current Knowledge of the Interrelationship Between Microbial Dysbiosis and Skin Conditions," 353.

4. Dora Hrestak et al, "Skin Microbiota in Atopic Dermatitis," *International Journal of Molecular Sciences* 23, no. 7 (2022): 3503.

5. Karolina Chilicka et al., "Microbiome and Probiotics in Acne Vulgaris—A Narrative Review," *Life* 12, no. 3 (2022): 422.

6. Jean-Paul Claudel et al., "*Staphylococcus epidermidis*: A Potential New Player in the Physiopathology of Acne?" *Dermatology* 235, no. 4 (2019): 287–94.

7. Pessemier et al., "Gut-Skin Axis: Current Knowledge of the Interrelationship Between Microbial Dysbiosis and Skin Conditions," 353.

8. Mariusz Sikora et al., "Gut Microbiome in Psoriasis: an Updated Review," *Pathogens* 9, no. 6 (2020): 463.

9. Silvia Carmona-Cruz, Luz Orozco-Covarrubias, and Marimar Sáez-de-Ocariz, "The Human Skin Microbiome in Selected Cutaneous Diseases," *Frontiers in Cellular and Infection Microbiology* 12 (2022): 834135.

10. Hei Sung Kim, "Microbiota in Rosacea," *American Journal of Clinical Dermatology* 21, no. Suppl 1 (2020): 25–35.

11. Rituja Saxena et al., "Comparison of Healthy and Dandruff Scalp Microbiome Reveals the Role of Commensals in Scalp Health," *Frontiers in Cellular and Infection Microbiology* 8 (2018): 346.

12. Qingbin Lin et al., "Malassezia and Staphylococcus Dominate Scalp Microbiome for Seborrheic Dermatitis," *Bioprocess and Biosystems Engineering* 44, no. 5 (2021): 965–75.

13. Brian Siu-Hin Ho et al., "Microbiome in the hair follicle of androgenetic alopecia patients," *PLoS One* 14, no. 5 (2019): e0216330.

14. Katarzyna Polak-Witka et al., "The Role of the Microbiome in Scalp Hair Follicle Biology and Disease," *Experimental Dermatology* 29, no. 3 (2020): 286–94.

15. Yu Ri Woo et al., "The Human Microbiota and Skin Cancer," *International Journal of Molecular Sciences* 23, no. 3 (2022): 1813.

16. Pessemier et al., "Gut-Skin Axis: Current Knowledge of the Interrelationship Between Microbial Dysbiosis and Skin Conditions," 353; "Harnessing the skin's microbiome could help combat skin aging," https://www.medicalnewstoday. com/articles/harnessing-the-skins-microbiome-could-help-combat-skin-aging

17. L. Gao et al, "Oral Microbiomes: More and More Importance in Oral Cavity and Whole Body," *Protein and Cell* 9, no. 5 (2018): 488–500; M. Kilian et al, "The Oral Microbiome – an Update for Oral Healthcare Professionals," *British Dental Journal* 221, no. 10 (2016): 657–66.

18. Lea Sedghi et al., "The Oral Microbiome: Role of Key Organisms and Complex Networks in Oral Health and Disease," *Periodontology 2000* 87, no. 1 (2021): 107–31.

19. Christina Kumpitsch et al., "The Microbiome of the Upper Respiratory Tract in Health and Disease," *BMC Biology* 17, no. 1 (2019): 87.

20. Samantha A. Whiteside, John E. McGinniss, and Ronald G. Collman, "The Lung Microbiome: Progress and Promise," *Journal of Clinical Investigation* 131, no. 15 (2021): e150473.

21. *Alzheimer's disease*: Dean M. Wingerchuk et al., "International Consensus Diagnostic Criteria for Neuromyelitis Optica Spectrum Disorders," *Neurology* 85, no. 2 (2015): 177–89; *Parkinson's disease*: Antje Haehner, Thomas Hummel, and Heinz Reichmann, "Olfactory Loss in Parkinson's Disease," *Parkinson's Disease* 2011 (2011): article ID 450939; *Covid*: Joaquim Mullol et al., "The Loss of Smell and Taste in the COVID-19 Outbreak: a Tale of Many Countries," *Current Allergy and Asthma Reports* 20, no. 10 (2020): 61.

22. 'Pulmonary medicine at GBMC,' https://www.gbmc.org/pulmonary

23. Saroj Khatiwada and Astha Subedi, "Lung Microbiome and Coronavirus Disease 2019 (COVID-19): Possible Link and Implications," *Human Microbiome Journal* 17 (2020): 100073.

24. Anh Thu Dang and Benjamin J. Marsland, "Microbes, Metabolites, and the Gut–Lung Axis," *Mucosal Immunology* 12, no. 4 (2019): 843–50.

Chapter 10

1. Jacques Ravel et al., "Vaginal Microbiome of Reproductive-Age Women," *Proceedings of the National Academy of Sciences of the United States of America* 108 Suppl. 1 (2011): 4680–7; Jessica S. Wells et al., "The Vaginal Microbiome in U. S. Black Women: A Systematic Review," *Journal of Women's Health* 29, no. 3 (2020): 362–75.

2. Harrisham Kaur et al., "Crosstalk Between Female Gonadal Hormones and Vaginal Microbiota Across Various Phases of Women's Gynecological Lifecycle," *Frontiers in Microbiology* 11 (2020): 551.

3. Yumna Moosa et al., "Determinants of Vaginal Microbiota Composition," *Frontiers in Cellular and Infection Microbiology* 10 (2020): 467.

4. Harrisham Kaur et al., "Crosstalk Between Female Gonadal Hormones and Vaginal Microbiota Across Various Phases of Women's Gynecological Lifecycle," *Frontiers in Microbiology* 11 (2020): 551; Emmanuel Amabebe and Dilly O. C. Anumba, "The Vaginal Microenvironment: the Physiologic Role of Lactobacilli," *Frontiers in Medicine* 5 (2018): 181.

5. Janneke H. H. M. van de Wijgert et al., "The Vaginal Microbiota: What Have We Learned After a Decade of Molecular Characterization?" *PLOS ONE* 9, no. 8 (2014): e105998.

6. Linda Abou Chacra, Florence Fenollar, and Khoudia Diop, "Bacterial Vaginosis: What Do We Currently Know?" *Frontiers in Cellular and Infection Microbiology* 11 (2021): 672429.

7. Xiaodi Chen et al., "The Female Vaginal Microbiome in Health and Bacterial Vaginosis," *Frontiers in Cellular and Infection Microbiology* 11 (2021): 631972.

8. Linda Abou Chacra, Florence Fenollar, and Khoudia Diop, "Bacterial Vaginosis: What Do We Currently Know?" *Frontiers in Cellular and Infection Microbiology* 11 (2021): 672429.

9. Xiaodi Chen et al., "The Female Vaginal Microbiome in Health and Bacterial Vaginosis," *Frontiers in Cellular and Infection Microbiology* 11 (2021): 631972.

10. Anjani Chandra, Casey E. Copen, and Elizabeth Hervey Stephen, "Infertility and Impaired Fecundity in the United States, 1982–2010: Data from the National Survey of Family Growth," *National Health Statistics Reports* 67, no. 67 (2013): 1–19.

11. Olivia Moumne et al., "Implications of the Vaginal Microbiome and Potential Restorative Strategies on Maternal Health: a Narrative Review," *Journal of Perinatal Medicine* 49, no. 4 (2021): 402–11; Salvatore Giovanni Vitale et al., "The Role of Genital Tract Microbiome in Fertility: A Systematic Review," *International Journal of Molecular Sciences* 23, no. 1 (2021): 180.

12. Inmaculada Moreno et al., "Evidence That the Endometrial Microbiota Has an Effect on Implantation Success or Failure," *American Journal of Obstetrics and Gynecology* 215, no. 6 (2016): 684–703.

13. Ruairi C. Robertson et al., "The Human Microbiome and Child Growth – First 1000 Days and Beyond," *Trends in Microbiology* 27, no. 2 (2019): 131–47.

14. Richard Cariño et al., "The Search for Aliens Within Us: A Review of Evidence and Theory Regarding the Foetal Microbiome," *Critical Reviews in Microbiology* 48, no. 5 (2022): 611–23; Archita Mishra et al., "Microbial Exposure During Early Human Development Primes Fetal Immune Cells," *Cell* 184, no. 13 (2021): 3394–3409.e20.

15. Sabrina Tamburini et al., "The Microbiome in Early Life: Implications for Health Outcomes," *Nature Medicine* 22, no. 7 (2016): 713–22.

16. Word Health Organization, "Breastfeeding," https://www.who.int/health-topics/breastfeeding#tab=tab_1

17. Lars Bode, "Human Milk Oligosaccharides: Every Baby Needs a Sugar Mama," *Glycobiology* 22, no. 9 (2012): 1147–62; Su Yeong Kim and Dae Yong Yi, "Components of Human Breast Milk: from Macronutrient to Microbiome and microRNA," *Clinical and Experimental Pediatrics* 63, no. 8 (2020): 301–9.

18. Shirin Moossavi et al., "Composition and Variation of the Human Milk Microbiota Are Influenced by Maternal and Early-Life Factors," *Cell Host and Microbe* 25, no. 2 (2019): 324–335.e4.

19. Modupe O. Coker et al., "Infant Feeding Alters the Longitudinal Impact of Birth Mode on the Development of the Gut Microbiota in the First Year of Life," *Frontiers in Microbiology* 12 (2021): [642197].

20. Erika Cortes-Macías et al., "Maternal Diet Shapes the Breast Milk Microbiota Composition and Diversity: Impact of Mode of Delivery and Antibiotic Exposure," *Journal of Nutrition* 151, no. 2 (2021): 330–40.

21. Eunice Kennedy Shriver National Institute of Child Health and Human Development, "What is weaning and how do I do it?" https://www.nichd.nih.gov/health/topics/breastfeeding/conditioninfo/weaning

22. Christopher J. Stewart et al., "Temporal Development of the Gut Microbiome in Early Childhood from the TEDDY Study," *Nature* 562, no. 7728 (2018): 583–8.

23. Shirin Moossavi, and Meghan B. Azad, "Origins of Human Milk Microbiota: New Evidence and Arising Questions," *Gut Microbes* 12, no. 1 (2020): 1667722.

24. Alain Cuna et al., "Dynamics of the Preterm Gut Microbiome in Health and Disease," *American Journal of Physiology. Gastrointestinal and Liver Physiology* 320, no. 4 (2021): G411–9; Jannie G. E. Henderickx et al., "The Preterm Gut Microbiota: an Inconspicuous Challenge in Nutritional Neonatal Care," *Frontiers in Cellular and Infection Microbiology* 9 (2019): 85.

25. Andrea C. Masi, and Christopher J. Stewart, "The Role of the Preterm Intestinal Microbiome in Sepsis and Necrotising Enterocolitis," *Early Human Development* 138 (2019): 104854.

26. Andrea C. Masi, and Christopher J. Stewart, "The Role of the Preterm Intestinal Microbiome in Sepsis and Necrotising Enterocolitis," *Early Human Development* 138 (2019): 104854; David J. Hackam and Chhinder P. Sodhi, "Bench to Bedside — New Insights into the Pathogenesis of Necrotizing Enterocolitis," *Nature Reviews. Gastroenterology and Hepatology* 19, no. 7 (2022): 468–79.

27. Christopher J. Stewart et al., "Temporal Bacterial and Metabolic Development of the Preterm Gut Reveals Specific Signatures in Health and Disease," *Microbiome* 4, no. 1 (2016): 67.

28. Kirsty Le Doare et al., "Mother's Milk: A Purposeful Contribution to the Development of the Infant Microbiota and Immunity," *Frontiers in Immunology* 9 (2018): 361.

29. J. Meinzen-Derr et al., "Role of Human Milk in Extremely Low Birth Weight Infants' Risk of Necrotizing Enterocolitis or Death," *Journal of Perinatology: Official Journal of the California Perinatal Association* 29, no. 1 (2009): 57–62.

30. Rebecca L. Morgan et al., "Probiotics Reduce Mortality and Morbidity in Preterm, Low-Birth-Weight Infants: A Systematic Review and Network Meta-analysis of Randomized Trials," *Gastroenterology* 159, no. 2 (2020): 467–80.

31. 'Predict premature births and improve outcomes for mothers and babies,' https://www.ultrasound.ai

Chapter 11

1. Miles Berger, John A. Gray, and Bryan L. Roth, "The Expanded Biology of Serotonin," *Annual Review of Medicine* 60 (2009): 355–66.

2. Jessica M. Yano et al, "Indigenous Bacteria from the Gut Microbiota Regulate Host Serotonin Biosynthesis," *Cell* 161, no. 2 (2015): 264–76.

3. Bruna Neroni et al, "Relationship Between Sleep Disorders and Gut Dysbiosis: What Affects What?" *Sleep Medicine* 87 (2021): 1–7; Robert P. Smith et al, "Gut Microbiome Diversity Is Associated with Sleep Physiology in Humans," *PLOS ONE* 14, no. 10 (2019): e0222394.

4. Christoph A. Thaiss et al., "A Day in the Life of the Meta-organism: Diurnal Rhythms of the Intestinal Microbiome and Its Host," *Gut Microbes* 6, no. 2 (2015): 137–42; Yufei Tian et al, "An Important Link Between the Gut Microbiota and the Circadian Rhythm: Imply for Treatments of Circadian Rhythm Sleep Disorder," *Food Science and Biotechnology* 31, no. 2 (2022): 155–64.

5. Reiner Jumpertz et al., "Energy-Balance Studies Reveal Associations Between Gut Microbes, Caloric Load, and Nutrient Absorption in Humans," *American Journal of Clinical Nutrition* 94, no. 1, (2011): 58–65.

6. Allana Collen, *10% Human: How Your Body's Microbes Hold the Key to Health and Happiness*, New York: Harperscollins Publishers, 2015

7. Reiner Jumpertz et al., "Energy-Balance Studies Reveal Associations Between Gut Microbes, Caloric Load, and Nutrient Absorption in Humans," *American Journal of Clinical Nutrition* 94, no. 1 (2011): 58–65.

8. Ruth E. Ley et al., "Microbial Ecology: Human Gut Microbes Associated with Obesity." *Nature* 444, no. 7122 (2006): 1022–3.

9. Judith Aron-Wisnewsky and Karine Clément, "The Gut Microbiome, Diet, and Links to Cardiometabolic and Chronic Disorders," *Nature Reviews. Nephrology* 12, no. 3 (2016): 169–81.

10. Kymberleigh A. Romano et al., "Intestinal Microbiota Composition Modulates Choline Bioavailability from Diet and Accumulation of the Proatherogenic Metabolite Trimethylamine-N-oxide," *mBio* 6, no. 2 (2015): e02481.

11. Ahmad Ud Din et al., "Amelioration of TMAO Through Probiotics and Its Potential Role in Atherosclerosis," *Applied Microbiology and Biotechnology* 103, no. 23–24 (2019): 9217–28.

12. Nina Vinot, "6 Reasons Aligned with Your Values to Include More Plants in Your Diet," Jan 17, 2021, https://www.chicagomanualofstyle.org/tools_citationguide/citation-guide-1.html

13. María Arnoriaga-Rodríguez et al., "Gut Bacterial ClpB-Like Gene Function Is Associated with Decreased Body Weight and a Characteristic Microbiota Profile," *Microbiome* 8, no. 1 (2020): 59. DOI: 10.1186/s40168-020-00837-6.

14. N. Tennoune et al., "Bacterial ClpB Heat-Shock Protein, an Antigen-Mimetic of the Anorexigenic Peptide α-MSH, at the Origin of Eating Disorders," *Translational Psychiatry* 4 (2014): e458.

15. Serguei O. Fetissov, "Role of the Gut Microbiota in Host Appetite Control: Bacterial Growth to Animal Feeding Behaviour," *Nature Reviews. Endocrinology* 13, no. 1 (2017): 11–25.

16. Romain Legrand et al, "Commensal Hafnia alvei strain Reduces Food Intake and Fat Mass in Obese Mice—a New Potential Probiotic for Appetite and Body

Weight Management," *International Journal of Obesity* 44, no. 5 (2020): 1041–51; Nicolas Lucas et al., "Hafnia alvei HA4597 Strain Reduces Food Intake and Body Weight Gain and Improves Body Composition, Glucose, and Lipid Metabolism in a Mouse Model of Hyperphagic Obesity," *Microorganisms* 8, no. 1 (2019): 35.

17. Pierre Déchelotte et al., "The Probiotic Strain H. alvei HA4597® Improves Weight Loss in Overweight Subjects Under Moderate Hypocaloric Diet: A Proof-of-Concept, Multicenter Randomized, Double-Blind Placebo-Controlled Study," *Nutrients* 13, no. 6 (2021).

18. Lawrence A. David et al., "Diet Rapidly and Reproducibly Alters the Human Gut Microbiome," *Nature* 505, no. 7484 (2014): 559–63.

19. Ruth E. Ley et al., "Microbial Ecology: Human Gut Microbes Associated with Obesity," *Nature* 444, no. 7122 (2006): 1022–3.

20. Nina Vinot, "Next Generation Probiotics," Mar 9, https://medium.com/illumination/next-generation-probiotics-ca973c28d6

21. Viviana Aya et al., "Association Between Physical Activity and Changes in Intestinal Microbiota Composition: A Systematic Review," *PLOS ONE* 16, no. 2 (2021): e0247039.

22. Nathalie Boisseau, Nicolas Barnich, and Christelle Koechlin-Ramonatxo, "The Nutrition-Microbiota-Physical Activity Triad: an Inspiring New Concept for Health and Sports Performance," *Nutrients* 14, no. 5 (2022): 924.

23. Alex E. Mohr et al, "The Athletic Gut Microbiota," *Journal of the International Society of Sports Nutrition* 17, no. 1 (2020): 24.

24. Ralf Jäger et al, "International Society of Sports Nutrition Position Stand: Probiotics," *Journal of the International Society of Sports Nutrition* 16, no. 1 (2019): 62; Riley L. Hughes, "A Review of the Role of the Gut Microbiome in Personalized Sports Nutrition," *Frontiers in Nutrition* 6 (2019): 191.

25. Philip A. Mackowiak, "Recycling Metchnikoff: Probiotics, the Intestinal Microbiome and the Quest for Long Life," *Frontiers in Public Health* 1 (2013): 52; Elie Methcnikoff, *The Prolongation of Life: Optimistic Studies*, London: William Heinemann, 1907, pp. 91–93.

26. Magda R. Hamczyk et al., "Biological Versus Chronological Aging: JACC Focus Seminar," *Journal of the American College of Cardiology* 75, no. 8 (2020): 919–30; Alexander M. Vaiserman, Alexander K. Koliada, and Francesco Marotta, "Gut Microbiota: A Player in Aging and a Target for Anti-aging Intervention," *Ageing Research Reviews* 35 (2017): 36–45.

27. Yuko Sato et al., "Novel Bile Acid Biosynthetic Pathways Are Enriched in the Microbiome of Centenarians," *Nature* 599, no. 7885 (2021): 458–64.

28. Alexander M. Vaiserman, Alexander K. Koliada, and Francesco Marotta, "Gut Microbiota: A Player in Aging and a Target for Anti-aging Intervention," *Ageing Research Reviews* 35 (2017): 36–45.

29. "Deep Longevity granted the first microbiomic aging clock patent," Press Release, July 6, 2022, https://www.eurekalert.org/news-releases/957936

30. Michael W. Gray, "Lynn Margulis and the endosymbiont hypothesis: 50 years later," *Molecular Biology of the Cell* 28, no. 10 (2017): 1285–7; Joseph Pizzorno, "Mitochondria-Fundamental to Life and Health," *Integrative Medicine* 13, no. 2 (2014): 8–15; Aleksandra Trifunovic, "Mitochondrial DNA and Ageing." *Biochimica et biophysica acta* 1757, no. 5–6 (2006): 611–7.

31. J. William O. Ballard and Samuel G. Towarnicki, "Mitochondria, the Gut Microbiome and ROS," *Cellular Signalling* 75 (2020): 109737.

Chapter 12

1. "Your gut . . . your health!" https://www.thegut.org.nz/resources/

2. Megan Cully, "Microbiome Therapeutics Go Small Molecule," *Nature Reviews. Drug Discovery* 18, no. 8 (2019): 569–72.

3. Ke Xiong et al., "Construction of food-grade pH-sensitive nanoparticles for delivering functional food ingredients," *Trends in Food Science & Technology* 96 (2020): 102–113.

Chapter 13

1. Robert W. Hutkins et al., "Prebiotics: Why Definitions Matter," *Current Opinion in Biotechnology* 37 (2016): 1–7.

2. "How Does Smoking Affect The Respiratory System?" http://www.rocketswag. com/medicine/anatomy/respiratory-system/How-Does-Smoking-Affect-The-Respiratory-System.html

3. Kunal Dixit et al., "Restoration of Dysbiotic Human Gut Microbiome for Homeostasis," *Life Sciences* 278: 119622.

4. Colin Hill et al, "Expert Consensus Document. The International Scientific Association for Probiotics and Prebiotics Consensus Statement on the Scope and Appropriate Use of the Term Probiotic," *Nature Reviews. Gastroenterology and Hepatology* 11, no. 8 (2014): 506–14.

5. "Probiotics and Prebiotics: the EU Ban Is Shaking: Some Countries Have Not Accepted the European Commission's Limitations on the Term 'Probiotic' and Have Implemented Their Own Interpretations," https://www.thefreeli-brary.com/Probiotics+%26+Prebiotics%3A+The+EU+Ban+is+Shaking%3A+Some+countries+have...-a0659376750.

6. Sabina Fijan, "Microorganisms with Claimed Probiotic Properties: an Overview of Recent Literature," *International Journal of Environmental Research and Public Health* 11, no. 5 (2014): 4745–67.

7. Yuqing Feng et al, "An Examination of Data from the American Gut Project Reveals That the Dominance of the Genus Bifidobacterium Is Associated with the Diversity and Robustness of the Gut Microbiota," *MicrobiologyOpen* 8, no. 12 (2019): e939.

8. Chyn Boon Wong, Toshitaka Odamaki, and Jin-Zhong Xiao, "Insights into the Reason of Human-Residential Bifidobacteria (HRB) Being the Natural Inhabitants of the Human Gut and Their Potential Health-Promoting Benefits," *FEMS Microbiology Reviews* 44, no. 3 (2020): 369–85.

9. Amy O'Callaghan, and Douwe van Sinderen, "Bifidobacteria and Their Role as Members of the Human Gut Microbiota," *Frontiers in Microbiology* 7 (2016): 925.

10. Tarini Shankar Ghosh, Jerome Arnoux, and Paul W. O'Toole, "Metagenomic Analysis Reveals Distinct Patterns of Gut Lactobacillus Prevalence, Abundance, and Geographical Variation in Health and Disease," *Gut Microbes* 12, no. 1 (2020): 1–19.

11. D. D. Heeney, M. G. Gareau, and M. L. Marco, "Intestinal Lactobacillus in Health and Disease, a Driver or Just Along for the Ride?" *Current Opinion in Biotechnology* 49 (2018): 140–7; Jacques Ravel et al, "Vaginal Microbiome of Reproductive-Age Women," *Proceedings of the National Academy of Sciences of the United States of America* 108 Suppl. 1 (2011): 4680–7; Floyd E. Dewhirst et al, "The Human Oral Microbiome," *Journal of Bacteriology* 192, no. 19 (2010): 5002–17.

12. Qinghui Mu, Vincent J. Tavella, and Xin M. Luo, "Role of Lactobacillus reuteri in Human Health and Diseases," *Frontiers in Microbiology* 9 (2018): 757.

13. H. Qi et al, "Lactobacillus Maintains Healthy Gut Mucosa by Producing L-ornithine," *Communications Biology* 2 (2019): 171.

14. Fouad M. F. Elshaghabee et al., "Bacillus as Potential Probiotics: Status, Concerns, and Future Perspectives," *Frontiers in Microbiology* 8 (2017): 1490.

15. Na-Kyoung Lee, Won-Suck Kim, and Hyun-Dong Paik, "Bacillus Strains as Human Probiotics: Characterization, Safety, Microbiome, and Probiotic Carrier," *Food Science and Biotechnology* 28, no. 5 (2019): 1297–305.

16. Paul W. O'Toole, Julian R. Marchesi, and Colin Hill, "Next-Generation Probiotics: the Spectrum from Probiotics to Live Biotherapeutics," *Nature Microbiology* 2 (2017): 17057.

17. Rebeca Martín, and Philippe Langella, "Emerging Health Concepts in the Probiotics Field: Streamlining the Definitions," *Frontiers in Microbiology* 10 (2019): 1047

18. Nina Vinot, "Next-Generation Probiotics," https://medium.com/illumination/next-generation-probiotics-ca973c28d6

19. "The Earth Microbiome Project is a systematic attempt to characterize global microbial taxonomic and functional diversity for the benefit of the planet and humankind," https://earthmicrobiome.org/

20. Glenn R. Gibson et al, "Expert Consensus Document: the International Scientific Association for Probiotics and Prebiotics (ISAPP) Consensus Statement on the Definition and Scope of Prebiotics," *Nature Reviews. Gastroenterology and Hepatology* 14, no. 8 (2017): 491–502.

21. Justin L. Carlson et al., "Health Effects and Sources of Prebiotic Dietary Fiber," *Current Developments in Nutrition* 2, no. 3 (2018): nzy005.

22. Hannah D. Holscher, "Dietary Fiber and Prebiotics and the Gastrointestinal Microbiota," *Gut Microbes* 8, no. 2 (2017): 172–84.

23. Joanne Slavin, "J. Fiber and Prebiotics: Mechanisms and Health Benefits," *Nutrients* 5, no. 4 (2013): 1417–35.

24. Kirsty Le Doare et al., "Mother's Milk: A Purposeful Contribution to the Development of the Infant Microbiota and Immunity," *Frontiers in Immunology* 9 (2018): 361.

25. Yvan Vandenplas et al, "Human Milk Oligosaccharides: 2'-Fucosyllactose (2'-FL) and Lacto-N-Neotetraose (LNnT) in Infant Formula," *Nutrients* 10, no. 9 (2018): 1161.

26. E. Elison et al, "Oral Supplementation of Healthy Adults with2'-O-fucosyllactose and Lacto-N-neotetraose Is Welltolerated and Shifts the Intestinal Microbiota," *British Journal of Nutrition* 116, no. 8 (2016): 1356–68.

27. Hannah Cory et al., "The Role of Polyphenols in Human Health and Food Systems: A Mini-Review," *Frontiers in Nutrition* 5 (2018): 87.

28. Kelly S. Swanson et al, "The International Scientific Association for Probiotics and Prebiotics (ISAPP) Consensus Statement on the Definition and Scope of Synbiotics," *Nature Reviews. Gastroenterology and Hepatology* 17, no. 11 (2020): 687–701.

29. Seppo Salminen et al, "The International Scientific Association of Probiotics and Prebiotics (ISAPP) Consensus Statement on the Definition and Scope of Postbiotics," *Nature Reviews. Gastroenterology and Hepatology* 18, no. 9 (2021): 649–67.

30. Arthur C. Ouwehand and S. J. Salminen, "The Health Effects of Cultured Milk Products with Viable and Non-viable Bacteria," *International Dairy Journal* 8, no. 9 (1998): 749–58.

31. Neslihan Yeşilyurt et al., "Involvement of Probiotics and Postbiotics in the Immune System Modulation," *Biologics* 1, no. 2 (2021): 89–110.

32. "What are probiotics?" https://isappscience.org/for-consumers/learn/probiotics/

33. Q. Hao, B. R. Dong, and T. Wu, "Probiotics for Preventing Acute Upper Respiratory Tract Infections," *Cochrane Database of Systematic Reviews* 2 (2015): CD006895; Fabrizio Pregliasco et al., "A New Chance of Preventing Winter Diseases by the Administration of Synbiotic Formulations," *Journal of Clinical Gastroenterology* 42 Suppl. 3 Pt 2 (2008): S224–33.

34. Hania Szajewska et al., "Probiotics for the Prevention of Antibiotic-Associated Diarrhea in Children," *Journal of Pediatric Gastroenterology and Nutrition* 62, no. 3 (2016): 495–506.

35. Mario Del Piano et al., "The Use of Probiotics in Healthy Volunteers with Evacuation Disorders and Hard Stools: a Double-Blind, Randomized,

Placebo-Controlled Study," *Journal of Clinical Gastroenterology* 44 Suppl. 1 (2010): S30–4; Eirini Dimidi, S. Mark Scott, and Kevin Whelan, "Probiotics and Constipation: Mechanisms of Action, Evidence for Effectiveness and Utilisation by Patients and Healthcare Professionals," *Proceedings of the Nutrition Society* 79, no. 1 (2020): 147–57.

36. Tina Didari et al., "Effectiveness of Probiotics in Irritable Bowel Syndrome: Updated Systematic Review with Meta-analysis," *World Journal of Gastroenterology* 21, no. 10 (2015): 3072–84; E. Arvidsson Nordström et al., "Lactiplantibacillus plantarum 299v (LP299V®): Three Decades of Research," *Beneficial Microbes* 12, no. 5 (2021): 441–65.

37. Pierre Déchelotte et al., "The Probiotic Strain H. alvei HA4597® Improves Weight Loss in Overweight Subjects Under Moderate Hypocaloric Diet: A Proof-of-Concept, Multicenter Randomized, Double-Blind Placebo-Controlled Study," *Nutrients* 13, no. 6 (2021): 1902; Simone Perna et al., "Is Probiotic Supplementation Useful for the Management of Body Weight and Other Anthropometric Measures in Adults Affected by Overweight and Obesity with Metabolic Related Diseases? A Systematic Review and Meta-analysis," Nutrients 13, no. 2 (2021): 666.

38. L. Drago et al., "Effects of Lactobacillus salivarius LS01 (DSM 22775) Treatment on Adult Atopic Dermatitis: a Randomized Placebo-Controlled Study," *International Journal of Immunopathology and Pharmacology* 24, no. 4 (2011): 1037–48; Alessandro Fiocchi et al, "World Allergy Organization-McMaster University Guidelines for Allergic Disease Prevention (GLAD-P): Probiotics," *World Allergy Organization Journal* 8, no. 1 (2015): 4; Carol Stephanie C. Tan-Lim et al., "Comparative Effectiveness of Probiotic Strains on the Prevention of Pediatric Atopic Dermatitis: A Systematic Review and Network Meta-analysis," *Pediatric Allergy and Immunology: Official Publication of the European Society of Pediatric Allergy and Immunology* 32, no. 6 (2021): 1255–70.

39. Azadeh Goodarzi et al., "The Potential of Probiotics for Treating Acne Vulgaris: A Review of Literature on Acne and Microbiota," *Dermatologic Therapy* 33, no. 3 (2020): e13279; A. M. Vargason and A. C. Anselmo, "Live Biotherapeutic Products and Probiotics for the Skin," *Advanced NanoBiomed Research* 1, no. 12 (2021): 2100118.

40. S. Atik et al."Efficacy of Probiotics Administration in Patients with Partly Controlled Asthma: A Randomized Placebo Controlled Trial," *Journal of Allergy and Clinical Immunology* 145, no. 2 (2020): AB19; Lorenzo Drago et al., "The Probiotics in Pediatric Asthma Management (PROPAM) Study in the Primary Care Setting: A Randomized, Controlled, Double-Blind Trial with Ligilactobacillus salivarius LS01 (DSM 22775) and Bifidobacterium breve B632 (DSM 24706)," *Journal of Immunology Research* 2022 (2022): 3837418.

41. Fraser L. Collins et al., "The Potential of Probiotics as a Therapy for Osteoporosis," *Microbiology Spectrum* 5, no. 4 (2017); Hanieh Malmir et al., "Probiotics as a New Regulator for Bone Health: A Systematic Review and Meta-analysis," *Evidence-Based Complementary and Alternative Medicine*: eCAM 2021 (2021): 3582989.

42. Li-Hao Cheng et al., "Psychobiotics in Mental Health, Neurodegenerative and Neurodevelopmental Disorders," *Journal of Food and Drug Analysis* 27, no. 3 (2019): 632–48; Richa Sharma et al., "Psychobiotics: the Next-Generation Probiotics for the Brain," *Current Microbiology* 78, no. 2 (2021): 449–63; https://cerebiomebylallemand.com

43. Leónides Fernández et al., "Application of Ligilactobacillus salivarius CECT5713 to Achieve Term Pregnancies in Women with Repetitive Abortion or Infertility of Unknown Origin by Microbiological and Immunological Modulation of the Vaginal Ecosystem," *Nutrients* 13, no. 1 (2021): 162.

44. N. M. de Roos et al., "The Effects of the Multispecies Probiotic Mixture Ecologic®Barrier on Migraine: Results of an Open-Label Pilot Study," *Beneficial Microbes* 6, no. 5 (2015): 641–6.

45. Melissa Barker et al., "Probiotics and Human Lactational Mastitis: A Scoping Review," *Women and Birth: Journal of the Australian College of Midwives* 33, no. 6 (2020): e483–91.

46. "Probiotics: A Role in Epilepsy?" https://www.teknoscienze.com/probiotics-a-role-in-epilepsy/

47. "Clinical Guide to Probiotic Products Available in USA," http://www.usprobioticguide.com/?utm_source=intro_pg&utm_medium=civ&utm_campaign=USA_CHART; "Clinical Guide to Probiotic Products Available in Canada," http://www.probioticchart.ca/?utm_source=intro_pg&utm_medium=civ&utm_campaign=CDN_CHART

48. "Infographics, Fact Sheets & Documents," https://internationalprobiotics.org/infographics/; "Infographics," https://isappscience.org/for-consumers/infographics/; "Know the Name of the Strain," http://www.aeprobio.com/infographics/

49. Colin Hill et al., "Expert Consensus Document. The International Scientific Association for Probiotics and Prebiotics Consensus Statement on the Scope and Appropriate Use of the Term Probiotic," *Nature Reviews. Gastroenterology and Hepatology* 11, no. 8 (2014): 506–14.

50. Sylvie Binda et al., "Criteria to Qualify Microorganisms as 'Probiotic' in Foods and Dietary Supplements," *Frontiers in Microbiology* 11 (2020): 1662.

51. EFSA Panel on Dietetic Products, Nutrition and Allergies (NDA), "Scientific Opinion on the substantiation of health claims related to live yoghurt cultures and improved lactose digestion (ID 1143, 2976) pursuant to Article 13(1) of Regulation (EC) No 1924/2006," *EFSA Journal* 2010, 8 (10): 1763.

52. Maria L. Marco et al., "Health Benefits of Fermented Foods: Microbiota and Beyond," *Current Opinion in Biotechnology* 44 (2017): 94–102; Maria L. Marco et

al, "The International Scientific Association for Probiotics and Prebiotics (ISAPP) Consensus Statement on Fermented Foods," *Nature Reviews. Gastroenterology and Hepatology* 18, no. 3 (2021): 196–208; Nevin Şanlier, Büşra Başar Gökcen, and Aybüke Ceyhun Sezgin, "Health Benefits of Fermented Foods," *Critical Reviews in Food Science and Nutrition* 59, no. 3 (2019): 506–27.

53. Marcel van de Wouw et al., "Distinct Actions of the Fermented Beverage Kefir on Host Behaviour, Immunity and Microbiome Gut-Brain Modules in the Mouse," *Microbiome* 8, no. 1 (2020): 67.

54. Jack A. Gilbert, Rob Knight, Sandra Blakeslee, *Dirt is Good: The Advantage of Germs for Your Child's Developing Immune System*, St. Martin's Press, 2017, https://www.goodreads.com/book/show/31450974-dirt-is-good

55. Seppo Salminen et al., "The International Scientific Association of Probiotics and Prebiotics (ISAPP) Consensus Statement on the Definition and Scope of Postbiotics," *Nature Reviews. Gastroenterology and Hepatology* 18, no. 9 (2021): 649–67.

56. José Eleazar Aguilar-Toalá et al., "Postbiotics — When Simplification Fails to Clarify," *Nature Reviews. Gastroenterology and Hepatology* 18, no. 11 (2021): 825–6; Seppo Salminen et al., "Reply to: Postbiotics – When Simplification Fails to Clarify," *Nature Reviews. Gastroenterology and Hepatology* 18, no. 11 (2021): 827–8.

57. Basavaprabhu H. Nataraj et al., "Postbiotics-Parabiotics: the New Horizons in Microbial Biotherapy and Functional Foods," *Microbial Cell Factories* 19, no. 1 (2020): 168.

58. Nina Vinot, "Did you miss Probiota Copenhagen 2022? Catch up now!" *Microbiome Times*, 12 April 2022, https://www.microbiometimes.com/did-you-miss-probiota-copenhagen-2022-catch-up-now/?utm_source=rss&utm_medium=rss&utm_campaign=did-you-miss-probiota-copenhagen-2022-catch-up-now

59. Ibid.

60. María José Hernández-Granados and Elena Franco-Robles, "Postbiotics in Human Health: Possible New Functional Ingredients?" *Food Research International* 137 (2020): 109660; P. F. Cuevas-González, A. M. Liceaga, and J. E. Aguilar-Toalá, "Postbiotics and Paraprobiotics: from Concepts to Applications," *Food Research International* 136 (2020): 109502.

61. Hang-Yu Li et al., "Effects and Mechanisms of Probiotics, Prebiotics, Synbiotics, and Postbiotics on Metabolic Diseases Targeting Gut Microbiota: A Narrative Review," *Nutrients* 13, no. 9 (2021): 3211.

62. P. F. Cuevas-González, A. M. Liceaga, and J. E. Aguilar-Toalá, "Postbiotics and Paraprobiotics: from Concepts to Applications," *Food Research International* 136 (2020): 109502.

63. EFSA Panel on Nutrition, Novel Foods and Food Allergens (NDA), Dominique Turck et al., "Safety of pasteurised Akkermansia muciniphila as a novel food

pursuant to Regulation (EU) 2015/2283," *EFSA journal. European Food Safety Authority* 19, no. 9 (2021): e06780

Chapter 14

1. Faming Zhang et al, "Microbiota Transplantation: Concept, Methodology and Strategy for Its Modernization," *Protein and Cell* 9, no. 5 (2018): 462–73; Faming Zhang et al., "Should We Standardize the 1,700-Year-Old Fecal Microbiota Transplantation?" *American Journal of Gastroenterology* 107, no. 11 (2012): 1755; author reply p. 1755–6; Jiunn-Wei Wang et al, "Fecal Microbiota Transplantation: Review and Update," *Journal of the Formosan Medical Association* 118 Suppl. 1 (2019): S23–S31.

2. Joshua Stripling, and Martin Rodriguez, "Current Evidence in Delivery and Therapeutic Uses of Fecal Microbiota Transplantation in Human Diseases—Clostridium difficile Disease and Beyond," *American Journal of the Medical Sciences* 356, no. 5 (2018): 424–32.

3. Joshua Stripling, and Martin Rodriguez, "Current Evidence in Delivery and Therapeutic Uses of Fecal Microbiota Transplantation in Human Diseases—Clostridium difficile Disease and Beyond," *American Journal of the Medical Sciences* 356, no. 5 (2018): 424–32; Howard Junca, Dietmar H. Pieper, and Eva Medina, "The Emerging Potential of Microbiome Transplantation on Human Health Interventions," *Computational and Structural Biotechnology Journal* 20 (2022): 615–27.

4. Howard Junca, Dietmar H. Pieper, and Eva Medina, "The Emerging Potential of Microbiome Transplantation on Human Health Interventions," *Computational and Structural Biotechnology Journal* 20 (2022): 615–27; E. M. Terveer et al, "How to: Establish and Run a Stool Bank," *Clinical Microbiology and Infection* 23, no. 12 (2017): 924–30; S. M. D. Baunwall et al, "The Use of Faecal Microbiota Transplantation (FMT) in Europe: A Europe-Wide Survey," *The Lancet Regional Health. Europe* 9 (2021): 100181.

5. Barbara H. McGovern et al, "SER-109, an Investigational Microbiome Drug to Reduce Recurrence After Clostridioides difficile Infection: Lessons Learned from a Phase 2 Trial," *Clinical Infectious Diseases* 72, no. 12 (2021): 2132–40.

6. Dongwen Ma, Yidan Chen, and Tingtao Chen, "Vaginal Microbiota Transplantation for the Treatment of Bacterial Vaginosis: a Conceptual Analysis," *FEMS Microbiology Letters* 366, no. 4 (2019).

7. Chris Callewaert et al., "Skin Microbiome Transplantation and Manipulation: Current State of the Art," *Computational and Structural Biotechnology Journal* 19 (2021): 624–31.

8. Dmitriy Myelnikov, "An Alternative Cure: the Adoption and Survival of Bacteriophage Therapy in the USSR, 1922–1955," *Journal of the History of*

Medicine and Allied Sciences 73, no. 4 (2018): 385–411; Karl Thiel, "Old Dogma, New Tricks—21st Century Phage Therapy," *Nature Biotechnology* 22, no. 1 (2004): 31–6; Richard Stone, "Bacteriophage Therapy. Stalin's Forgotten Cure," *Science* 298, no. 5594 (2002): 728–31; George Eliava (1892–1937), https://en.wikipedia.org/wiki/George_Eliava

9. Luis F. Camarillo-Guerrero et al., "Massive Expansion of Human Gut Bacteriophage Diversity," *Cell* 184, no. 4 (2021): 1098–1109.e9.

10. Marialetizia Rastelli, Claude Knauf, and Patrice D. Cani, "Gut Microbes and Health: A Focus on the Mechanisms Linking Microbes, Obesity, and Related Disorders," *Obesity* 26, no. 5 (2018): 792–800.

11. Ramy K. Aziz et al., "Translating Pharmacomicrobiomics: Three Actionable Challenges/Prospects in 2020," *Omics* 24, no. 2 (2020): 60–1.

12. Dan M. Roden et al., "Pharmacogenomics: the Genetics of Variable Drug Responses," *Circulation* 123, no. 15 (2011): 1661–70.

13. Concetta Panebianco, Angelo Andriulli, and Valerio Pazienza, "Pharmacomicrobiomics: Exploiting the Drug-Microbiota Interactions in Anticancer Therapies," *Microbiome* 6, no. 1 (2018): 92.

14. Les Dethlefsen and David A. Relman, "Incomplete Recovery and Individualized Responses of the Human Distal Gut Microbiota to Repeated Antibiotic Perturbation," *Proceedings of the National Academy of Sciences of the United States of America* 108 Suppl. 1 Suppl. 1(Suppl 1), 4554–4561 (2011): 4554–61.

15. Lisa Maier et al., "Extensive Impact of Non-antibiotic Drugs on Human Gut Bacteria," *Nature* 555, no. 7698 (2018): 623–8.

16. Matthew A. Jackson et al., "Gut Microbiota Associations with Common Diseases and Prescription Medications in a Population-Based Cohort," *Nature Communications* 9, no. 1 (2018): 2655.

17. Jacobo de la Cuesta-Zuluaga et al, "Metformin Is Associated with Higher Relative Abundance of Mucin-Degrading Akkermansia Muciniphila and Several Short-Chain Fatty Acid-Producing Microbiota in the Gut," *Diabetes Care* 40, no. 1 (2017): 54–62.

18. Elaine F. Enright et al., "The Impact of the Gut Microbiota on Drug Metabolism and Clinical Outcome," *Yale Journal of Biology and Medicine* 89, no. 3 (2016): 375–82.

19. Rosina Pryor et al., "The Role of the Microbiome in Drug Response," *Annual Review of Pharmacology and Toxicology* 60, no. 1 (2020): 417–35.

20. Sebastiaan P. van Kessel et al, "Gut Bacterial Tyrosine Decarboxylases Restrict Levels of Levodopa in the Treatment of Parkinson's Disease," *Nature Communications* 10, no. 1 (2019): 310.

21. Padmanee Sharma et al., "Primary, Adaptive, and Acquired Resistance to Cancer Immunotherapy," *Cell* 168, no. 4 (2017): 707–23.

22. V. Gopalakrishnan et al, "Gut Microbiome Modulates Response to Anti-PD-1 Immunotherapy in Melanoma Patients," *Science* 359, no. 6371 (2018): 97–103.

23. Yiming Wang et al., "Modulation of Gut Microbiota: A Novel Paradigm of Enhancing the Efficacy of Programmed death-1 and Programmed Death ligand-1 Blockade Therapy," *Frontiers in Immunology* 9 (MAR) (2018): 374.

24. Marwah Doestzada et al, "Pharmacomicrobiomics: a Novel Route Towards Personalized Medicine?" *Protein and Cell* 9, no. 5 (2018): 432–45.

25. Rosina Pryor et al., "The Role of the Microbiome in Drug Response," *Annual Review of Pharmacology and Toxicology* 60, no. 1 (2020): 417–35.

26. Giandomenico Roviello et al., "The Gut Microbiome and Efficacy of Cancer Immunotherapy," *Pharmacology and Therapeutics* 231 (2022): 107973.

27. Jessica Vamathevan et al, "Applications of Machine Learning in Drug Discovery and Development," *Nature Reviews. Drug Discovery* 18, no. 6 (2019): 463–77.

28. David J. Newman, and Gordon M. Cragg, "Natural Products as Sources of New Drugs over the Nearly Four Decades from 01/1981 to 09/2019," *Journal of Natural Products* 83, no. 3 (2020): 770–803.

29. K. A. Shaaban et al, "Pyramidamycins A-D and 3-Hydroxyquinoline-2-Carboxamide; Cytotoxic Benzamides from Streptomyces sp. DGC1," *Journal of Antibiotics* 65, no. 12 (2012): 615–22.

30. Laura E. McCoubrey et al., "Harnessing Machine Learning for Development of Microbiome Therapeutics," *Gut Microbes* 13, no. 1 (2021): 1–20.

Chapter 15

1. FDA-NIH Biomarker Working Group and BEST, "(Biomarkers, EndpointS, and Other Tools) Resource [Internet]," Silver Spring, (MD): Food and Drug Administration. US (2016–), https://www.ncbi.nlm.nih.gov/books/NBK326791/ Co-published by National Institutes of Health (US). Bethesda, (MD).

2. Khalid Saad Alharbi et al, "Gut Microbiota Disruption in COVID-19 or Post-COVID Illness Association with Severity Biomarkers: A Possible Role of Pre/Pro-biotics in Manipulating Microflora," *Chemico-Biological Interactions* 358 (2022): 109898.

3. Claire M. Doocey et al., "The Impact of the Human Microbiome in Tumorigenesis, Cancer Progression, and Biotherapeutic Development," *BMC Microbiology* 22, no. 1 (2022): 53.

4. Rongrong Li, Jilu Shen, and Yuanhong Xu, "Fusobacterium nucleatum and Colorectal Cancer," *Infection and Drug Resistance* 15 (2022): 1115–20.

5. Leonardo Mancabelli et al, "Identification of Universal Gut Microbial Biomarkers of Common Human Intestinal Diseases by Meta-analysis," *FEMS Microbiology Ecology* 93, no. 12 (2017).

6. Angelica Varesi et al, "The Potential Role of Gut Microbiota in Alzheimer's Disease: from Diagnosis to Treatment," *Nutrients* 14, no. 3 (2022): 668; Diana Marcela Mejía-Granados et al, "Gut Microbiome in Neuropsychiatric Disorders,"

Arquivos de Neuro-Psiquiatria 80, no. 2 (2022): 192–207; Kurumi Taniguchi et al., "D-Amino Acids as a Biomarker in Schizophrenia," *Diseases* 10, no. 1 (2022): 9; Sara Gerhardt and M. Hasan Mohajeri, "Changes of Colonic Bacterial Composition in Parkinson's Disease and Other Neurodegenerative Diseases," *Nutrients* 10, no. 6 (2018): 708; Lucía N. Peralta-Marzal et al, "The Impact of Gut Microbiota-Derived Metabolites in Autism Spectrum Disorders," *International Journal of Molecular Sciences* 22, no. 18 (2021): 10052.

7. Giandomenico Roviello et al., "The Gut Microbiome and Efficacy of Cancer Immunotherapy," *Pharmacology and Therapeutics* 231 (2022): 107973.

8. Tamara Glyn and Rachel Purcell, "Circulating Bacterial DNA: A New Paradigm for Cancer Diagnostics," *Frontiers in Medicine* 9 (2022): 831096.

9. Dan Knights et al., "Human-Associated Microbial Signatures: Examining Their Predictive Value," *Cell Host and Microbe* 10, no. 4 (2011): 292–6.

10. Ibid.

11. Bárbara Costa and Nuno Vale, "Drug Metabolism for the Identification of Clinical Biomarkers in Breast Cancer," *International Journal of Molecular Sciences* 23, no. 6 (2022): 3181.

12. G. Banavar et al, "The Salivary Metatranscriptome as an Accurate Diagnostic Indicator of Oral Cancer". https://www.researchsquare.com/article/rs-55052/v1 (2020).

13. Jake M. Robinson et al., "Forensic Applications of Microbiomics: A Review," *Frontiers in Microbiology* 11 (2020): 608101.

Chapter 16

1. Edward S. Chambers et al., "Role of Gut Microbiota-Generated Short-Chain Fatty Acids in Metabolic and Cardiovascular Health," *Current Nutrition Reports* 7, no. 4 (2018): 198–206.

2. Nathalie Boisseau, Nicolas Barnich, and Christelle Koechlin-Ramonatxo, "The Nutrition-Microbiota-Physical Activity Triad: an Inspiring New Concept for Health and Sports Performance," *Nutrients* 14, no. 5 (2022): 924.

3. Robert Caesar et al., "Crosstalk Between Gut Microbiota and Dietary Lipids Aggravates WAT Inflammation Through TLR Signaling," *Cell Metabolism* 22, no. 4 (2015): 658–68.

4. Viviana Aya et al., "Association Between Physical Activity and Changes in Intestinal Microbiota Composition: A Systematic Review," *PLOS ONE* 16, no. 2 (2021): e0247039.

5. J. Zhao et al., "Dietary Protein and Gut Microbiota Composition and Function," *CPPS* 20 (2018): 145–54.

6. Nathalie Boisseau, Nicolas Barnich, and Christelle Koechlin-Ramonatxo, "The Nutrition-Microbiota-Physical Activity Triad: an Inspiring New Concept for Health and Sports Performance," *Nutrients* 14, no. 5 (2022): 924; Saba Imdad et

al., "Intertwined Relationship of Mitochondrial Metabolism, Gut Microbiome and Exercise Potential," *International Journal of Molecular Sciences* 23, no. 5 (2022): 2679.

7. Lucy Mailing, "A comprehensive guide to stool and microbiome testing," June 2018, https://www.lucymailing.com/a-comprehensive-guide-to-stool-and-microbiome-testing/

8. "Human Genome Project," https://en.wikipedia.org/wiki/Human_Genome_Project

9. https://www.dnafit.com/; "Nutrition Report," https://genomelink.io/product/nutrition-advice-dna-report?gclid=Cj0KCQjw6J-SBhCrARIsAH0yMZhdxpKP-5wTkYpFssaadnUFkZBzwjbfi2_sbwui-E9s1fEnxjfEAELQaAk7ZEALw_wcB

10. https://www.daytwo.com/

11. Helena Mendes-Soares et al., "Assessment of a Personalized Approach to Predicting Postprandial Glycemic Responses to Food Among Individuals Without Diabetes," *JAMA Network Open* 2, no. 2 (2019): e188102; David Zeevi et al., "Personalized Nutrition by Prediction of Glycemic Responses," *Cell* 163, no. 5 (2015): 1079–94.

12. David Zeevi et al., "Personalized Nutrition by Prediction of Glycemic Responses," *Cell* 163, no. 5 (2015): 1079–94; "Blood Sugar Levels in Response to Foods Are Highly Individual," https://wis-wander.weizmann.ac.il/life-sciences/blood-sugar-levels-response-foods-are-highly-individual

13. Leonie Elizabeth et al., "Ultra-Processed Foods and Health Outcomes: A Narrative Review," *Nutrients* 12, no. 7 (2020): 1955; Mark L. Wahlqvist, "Regional Food Diversity and Human Health," *Asia Pacific Journal of Clinical Nutrition* 12, no. 3 (2003): 304–8.

14. Jacky Abitbol, Costanza Carissimo, and Vincent Sebag, "Behind the Term Sheet: How DayTwo is Revolutionizing Diabetes Care and Beyond with Microbiome Precision Nutrition," *Cathay Innovation*, 5 August 2021, https://medium.com/cathay-innovation/behind-the-term-sheet-how-daytwo-is-revolutionizing-diabetes-care-and-beyond-with-microbiome-dc944bbee407

15. National Institute of Diabetes and Digestive and Kidney Diseases, "Digestive Diseases Statistics for the United States," https://www.niddk.nih.gov/health-information/health-statistics/digestive-diseases

16. National Institutes of Health, "NIH Human Microbiome Project defines normal bacterial makeup of the body," 13 June 2012, https://www.nih.gov/news-events/news-releases/nih-human-microbiome-project-defines-normal-bacterial-makeup-body

Chapter 17

1. S. E. Adams et al., "A Randomised Clinical Study to Determine the Effect of a Toothpaste Containing Enzymes and Proteins on Plaque Oral Microbiome Ecology," *Scientific Reports* 7, no. 1 (2017): 43344.

Chapter 18

1. Barbara Cavalazzi et al, "Cellular Remains in a ~3.42-Billion-Year-Old Subseafloor Hydrothermal Environment," *Science Advances* 7, no. 29 (2021): eabf3963.
2. R. Brightman, "R. Perkin and the Dyestuffs Industry in Britain," *Nature* 177, no. 4514 (1956): 815–21.
3. Nitzan Koppel, Vayu Maini Rekdal, and Emily P. Balskus, "Chemical Transformation of Xenobiotics by the Human Gut Microbiota," *Science* 356, no. 6344 (2017): eaag2770.
4. Nitzan Koppel, Vayu Maini Rekdal, and Emily P. Balskus, "Chemical Transformation of Xenobiotics by the Human Gut Microbiota," *Science* 356, no. 6344 (2017): eaag2770.
5. Moddassir Ahmed et al., "Excessive Use of Nitrogenous Fertilizers: an Unawareness Causing Serious Threats to Environment and Human Health," *Environmental Science and Pollution Research International* 24, no. 35 (2017): 26983–7; Anna Engemann, Christine Focke, and Hans-Ulrich Humpf, "Intestinal Formation of N -Nitroso Compounds in the Pig Cecum Model," *Journal of Agricultural and Food Chemistry* 61, no. 4 (2013): 998–1005.
6. Ki-Hyun Kim, Ehsanul Kabir, and Shamin Ara Jahan, "Exposure to Pesticides and the Associated Human Health Effects," *Science of the Total Environment* 575 (2017): 525–35.
7. Xianling Yuan et al, "Gut Microbiota: an Underestimated and Unintended Recipient for Pesticide-Induced Toxicity," *Chemosphere* 227 (2019): 425–34.
8. Nitzan Koppel, Vayu Maini Rekdal, and Emily P. Balskus, "Chemical Transformation of Xenobiotics by the Human Gut Microbiota," *Science* 356, no. 6344 (2017): eaag2770.
9. Cheryl Qian Ying Yong, Suresh Valiyaveettil, and Bor Luen Tang, "Toxicity of Microplastics and Nanoplastics in Mammalian Systems," *International Journal of Environmental Research and Public Health* 17, no. 5 (2020): 1509.
10. R. Hampl, and L. Stárka, "Endocrine Disruptors and Gut Microbiome Interactions," *Physiological Research* 69, no. Suppl 2 (2020): S211–23. DOI: 10.33549/physiolres.934513.
11. Sayed Esmaeil Mousavi et al., "Air Pollution and Endocrine Disruptors Induce Human Microbiome Imbalances: A Systematic Review of Recent Evidence and

Possible Biological Mechanisms," *Science of the Total Environment* 816 (2022): 151654.

12. Stephanie L. Schnorr et al, "Gut Microbiome of the Hadza Hunter-Gatherers," *Nature Communications* 5 (2014): 3654; Jose C. Clemente et al, "The Microbiome of Uncontacted Amerindians," *Science Advances* 1, no. 3 (2015): e1500183.

13. M. P. Francino, "Antibiotics and the Human Gut Microbiome: Dysbioses and Accumulation of Resistances," *Frontiers in Microbiology* 6 (2015): 1543.

14. Paolo De Paoli, "Bio-banking in Microbiology: from Sample Collection to Epidemiology, Diagnosis and Research," *FEMS Microbiology Reviews* 29, no. 5 (2005): 897–910. DOI: 10.1016/j.femsre.2005.01.005.

15. N. E. Klepeis et al., "The National Human Activity Pattern Survey (NHAPS): a Resource for Assessing Exposure to Environmental Pollutants," *Journal of Exposure Analysis and Environmental Epidemiology* 11, no. 3 (2001): 231–52.

16. Alina Shrourou, "The Human Microbiome – A New Potential Fingerprint in Forensic Evidence?" An interview with Prof. Jack Gilbert, March 29, 2018, https://www.news-medical.net/news/20180329/The-Human-Microbiome-A-New-Potential-Fingerprint-in-Forensic-Evidence.aspx

17. Simon Lax et al., "Longitudinal Analysis of Microbial Interaction Between Humans and the Indoor Environment," *Science* (New York, NY) 345, no. 6200 (2014): 1048–52.

18. National Academies of Sciences, Engineering, and Medicine, *Microbiomes of the Built Environment: A Research Agenda for Indoor Microbiology, Human Health, and Buildings*, Washington, DC: The National Academies Press, 2017.

19. Martyn Dade-Robertson et al., "Architects of Nature: Growing Buildings with Bacterial Biofilms," *Microbial Biotechnology* 10, no. 5 (2017): 1157–63.

20. Vitruvius, *On Architecture*, Volume I: Books 1-5, Translated by Frank Granger, Loeb Classical Library 251, Cambridge, MA: Harvard University Press, 1931.

21. https://www.ioanaman.com/architecture-by-exposome

22. https://www.homebiotic.com; https://betterairus.com/

23. Jack A. Gilbert, Rob Knight, and Sandra Blakeslee, *Dirt is Good: The Advantage of Germs for Your Child's Developing Immune System*, St. Martin's Press, 2017.

24. Dr Qing Li, *Shinrin-Yoku: The Art and Science of Forest Bathing*, Penguin Life, 2018; Philip H. Siebler et al., "Acute Administration of the Nonpathogenic, Saprophytic Bacterium, Mycobacterium vaccae, Induces Activation of Serotonergic Neurons in the Dorsal Raphe Nucleus and Antidepressant-Like Behavior in Association with Mild Hypothermia," *Cellular and Molecular Neurobiology* 38, no. 1 (2018): 289–304; Dorothy M. Matthews, and Susan M. Jenks, "Ingestion of Mycobacterium vaccae Decreases Anxiety-Related Behavior and Improves Learning in Mice," *Behavioural Processes* 96 (2013): 27–35; James E. Hassell Jr. et al., "Treatment with a Heat-Killed Preparation of *Mycobacterium vaccae* After Fear Conditioning Enhances Fear Extinction

in the Fear-Potentiated Startle Paradigm," *Brain, Behavior, and Immunity* 81 (2019): 151–60.

25. Tove Fall et al., "Early Exposure to Dogs and Farm Animals and the Risk of Childhood Asthma," *JAMA Pediatrics* 169, no. 11 (2015): e153219.

26. Iona Mann, "The Architectural Exposome," https://static1.squarespace.com/static/5d29c446bd339b00010bed73/t/5e388f8e43b2a6137cb1e386/1580765080564/AArchitecture+37+Recognition_Exposome.pdf

27. Susan E. Coffin and Keith H. St. John, "Infection Control for Pediatric Hospitalists," in *Comprehensive Pediatric Hospital Medicine*, eds. Lisa B. Zaoutis, Vincent W. Chiang, Marylands Heights, Missouri: Mosby, 2007, pp. 28-31; Benedetta Allegranzi et al., "Burden of Endemic Health-Care-Associated Infection in Developing Countries: Systematic Review and Meta-analysis," *Lancet* 377, no. 9761 (2011): 228–41.

28. Hong Wang et al., "Probiotic Approach to Pathogen Control in Premise Plumbing Systems? A Review," *Environmental Science and Technology* 47, no. 18 (2013): 10117–28.

29. E. Caselli, P. Antonioli, and S. Mazzacane, "Safety of Probiotics Used for Hospital Environmental Sanitation," *Journal of Hospital Infection* 94, no. 2 (2016): 193–4.

30. Alberta Vandini et al., "Hard Surface Biocontrol in Hospitals Using Microbial-Based Cleaning Products," *PLOS ONE* 9, no. 9 (2014): e108598.

31. Elisabetta Caselli et al., "Impact of a Probiotic-Based Cleaning Intervention on the Microbiota Ecosystem of the Hospital Surfaces: Focus on the Resistome Remodulation," *PLOS ONE* 11, no. 2 (2016): e0148857.

32. World Health Organization, "Antimicrobial resistance," November 17, 2021, https://www.who.int/news-room/fact-sheets/detail/antimicrobial-resistance

33. Elisabetta Caselli et al., "Reducing Healthcare-Associated Infections Incidence by a Probiotic-Based Sanitation System: A Multicentre, Prospective, Intervention Study," *PLOS ONE* 13, no. 7 (2018): e0199616; Elisabetta Caselli, "Infezioni Ospedaliere: Prevenzione Con Probiotici E Fagi," https://microbioma.it/video/live-streaming/elisabetta-caselli-microbiologa-live-08-05-20/

34. Steven W. Kembel et al., "Architectural Design Influences the Diversity and Structure of the Built Environment Microbiome," *ISME Journal* 6, no. 8 (2012): 1469–79.

35. World Health Organization (WHO), "Worldwide country situation analysis: response to antimicrobial resistance," Summary, April 2015.

36. "Antimicrobial Resistance: Tackling a Crisis for the Health and Wealth of Nations," Review on Antimicrobial Resistance Chaired by Jim O'Neill, London, 2014.

37. Becky Little, "When London Faced a Pandemic—And a Devastating Fire," History.com, March 25, 2020, https://www.history.com/news/plague-pandemic-great-fire

38. Kat Springer, "Meet Luigi: MIT's sewer-scouring robot," *CNN Tech*, September 30, 2016, https://money.cnn.com/2016/09/30/technology/mit-robots-sewers/index.html

39. Cary Goldberg and Janet Wu, "MIT Offshoot That Detects Virus in Wastewater Raises $20 Million," *Bloomberg*, October 22, 2021, https://www.bloomberg.com/news/articles/2021-10-22/mit-offshoot-that-detects-virus-in-wastewater-raises-20-million?leadSource=uverify%20wall

40. Ethan D. Evans et al., "Longitudinal Wastewater Sampling in Buildings Reveals Temporal Dynamics of Metabolites," *PLOS Computational Biology* 16, no. 6 (2020 June 29): e1008001.

Chapter 19

1. U. S. Food and Drug Administration, "Early Clinical Trials with Live Biotherapeutic Products: Chemistry, Manufacturing, and Control Information," (FDA, 2016).

2. Iris Case, "The Regulation of Probiotics," *Writing Competition of John Hopkins University* (2021); Luis Gosálbez and Daniel Ramón, "Probiotics in Transition: Novel Strategies," *Trends in Biotechnology* 33, no. 4 (2015): 195–6.

3. Seppo Salminen et al, "The International Scientific Association of Probiotics and Prebiotics (ISAPP) Consensus Statement on the Definition and Scope of Postbiotics," *Nature Reviews. Gastroenterology and Hepatology* 18, no. 9 (2021): 649–67.

4. Meenu N. Perera et al., "Bacteriophage Cocktail Significantly Reduces or Eliminates Listeria monocytogenes Contamination on Lettuce, Apples, Cheese, Smoked Salmon and Frozen Foods," *Food Microbiology* 52 (2015): 42–8.

5. Arunava Kali, "Human Microbiome Engineering: the Future and Beyond," *Journal of Clinical and Diagnostic Research* 9, no. 9 (2015): DE01–4.

Epilogue

1. Ron Sender, Shai Fuchs, and Ron Milo, "Revised Estimates for the Number of Human and Bacteria Cells in the Body," *PLOS Biology* 14, no. 8 (2016): e1002533; Jack A. Gilbert et al, "Current Understanding of the Human Microbiome," *Nature Medicine* 24, no. 4 (2018): 392–400;

2. Tobias Rees, Thomas Bosch, and Angela E. Douglas, "How the Microbiome Challenges Our Concept of Self," *PLOS Biology* 16, no. 2 (2018): e2005358.

ABOUT THE AUTHORS

LEAD AUTHOR: Vladimir Jakovljevic, PhD

Vladimir is a molecular microbiologist with more than twenty years of experience. Throughout his research career, with teams of world-class scientists, Vladimir explored fundamental questions such as the structure and function of microbiomes, mechanisms of microbial virulence, motility and sensing of environmental signals. He is the author and co-author of numerous highly-cited publications and a contributor to various projects, as a scientific expert and as a project manager. Since 2020, Vladimir is the founder and owner of Microbiome Power (www.microbiomepower.com), a company dedicated to promotion of applications in the rapidly growing field of microbiome research.

Debojyoti Dhar, PhD

Dr Debojyoti Dhar, PhD is the co-founder and Director of South Asia's first microbiome company, Leucine Rich Bio Pvt Ltd. He received his PhD in molecular biology from the Indian Institute of Science (IISc) and has post-doctoral research experience from

UMass Medical School, USA. He has worked extensively on translational control of gene regulation during his PhD and post-doctoral research tenure. He has over fifteen years of experience in academic and industry 'research and development' (R&D) activities especially in metabolic syndrome, type 2 diabetes and gut health along with a strong multi domain expertise in pharmaceutical and biotechnology industries. He has held leadership positions in various companies with roles in R&D, Business Development, Corporate Communications and Consultancy and has thorough knowledge on new cutting-edge technologies in the bio-science space. An avid reader with aa keen interest in quantum physics and holistic medicine, Dr Dhar writes on disease, research and its impact on society and life science industry in general on his blog (www.debiisc.blogspot.in). Dr Dhar has to his credit various publications in top-tiered peer-reviewed scientific journals and is an active reviewer of scientific papers in many journals. He has co-authored a book-I, Microbiome meant for general reading apart from co-authoring other scientific books. Dr Dhar has been invited as a guest/keynote speaker at many conferences and institutes. He has also been featured in many science-based talk shows on various television channels such as German DW TV and Doordarshan (India). His interviews have also appeared in many media outlets such as, *The Economic Times*', *ET Prime*, *Indian Express*, *The Hindu Business Line*, *Chronicle PharmaBiz*, the *Times of India*, etc. Dr Dhar has led Leucine Rich Bio to win many national and international awards including the prestigious National Start-up award 2021, constituted by the Government of India.

Edda Russo, PhD

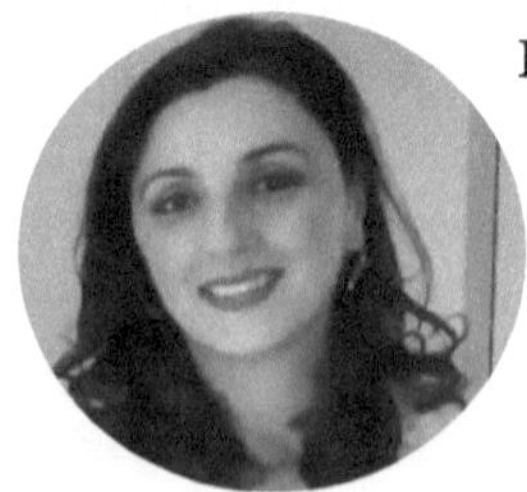

Edda graduated in 2006 with full marks and honours in Biology at Florence University. In 2012, she obtained the title of PhD in Biochemistry and Applied Biology. In 2021 she specialised in Clinical Pathology and Clinical Biochemistry with full marks and honours.

She works at the laboratory of Microbiome and Host Immunity, Department of Experimental and Clinical Medicine, University of Florence. She is the laboratory manager of the European project 'AMBROSIA', and is also a scientific grant writer, having done national and international collaborations. Her topic is the mutual interplay between the microbiome and immune response in several diseases and health conditions.

Her international profile is documented by scientific production: forty-two peer-reviewed articles, four book chapters". (see: ResearchGate).

Amedeo Amedei, PhD

Prof. Amedei graduated in 1996 with first-class honours in Biology at Florence University. He started his scientific career studying the role of Th1/Th2 lymphocytes in GVHD, atopic dermatitis and kidney rejection. Thereafter, he examined the role of *Helicobacter pylori*-specific immune response in gastric diseases. In 2003, he began his doctor's degree in 'Clinical and Experimental Medicine'. In 2005, he became a researcher at the Department of Experimental and Clinical Medicine, University of Florence, where in 2015 he was appointed as an Associate Professor.

Recently, Prof. Amedei has focused his scientific interests on cancer immunology and the role of the microbiome. The quality of his international profile is documented by his scientific production: 198 peer-reviewed articles (h-index: 54 and 9,627 Citations), seven book chapters and one patent (see: ResearchGate).

Prof. Amedei serves as an editorial board member of thirty international journals, as a Referee of forty-three Journals, and as a Co-Editor-Chief of one Journal. He carries out activities as a scientific reviewer for international research projects of private and public entities. Since 2016, he is in the Scientific Council of 'Toscana Life Sciences' (TLS). Till date, he has received more than € 6 million through proposals funded by several funding agencies, including the European Commission, Italian Ministry of Health, Tuscany Region, NASA, and several other local and international Foundations.

Aruna Rajan

Aruna Rajan, founder of Arogyam, has about two decades of experience helping companies in the healthcare sector make strategic decisions and accelerate, Return on Investment (ROI) through guided assessments. Prior to Arogyam, Aruna worked in the market insights group at Illumina, conducting market and competitive analyses to support senior executives for product marketing, investor relations, and sales. Before her stint at Illumina, Aruna was a strategy consultant at Scientia Advisors, a boutique life science strategy consulting company.

Her primary expertise lies in providing strategic insights and active information to life science companies along with lead problem-solving efforts by identifying issues, forming hypotheses, designing, and conducting analyses, and synthesizing conclusions into recommendations.

Nina Vinot

Nina is an enthusiast of symbioses and micro-organisms and is on a personal mission to spread the good word on the powers of bacteria. Co-chair of the International Probiotics Association Education and Communication Committee, lead of the Consumer Taskforce, member of the scientific advisory board of Agro Food Hi-Tech and a Bacterial blogger where she's an eager translator of the science jargon to business and to the public.

Nina's background is scientific. She holds an engineering master's in Agronomy from AgroParisTech, the leading school for life sciences in France where she specialized in nutrition. She was involved in the research of human and mice lemur nutrition at Penn State University, USA, the French National Center for Scientific Research (CNRS), and the National Institute for Agronomic Research (now INRAe).

Her experience in the nutraceuticals industry includes six years of successful development of probiotic supplements sales, technical marketing, and training of the sales force and distributors for Probiotical in Europe and totals about 10 years of technical sales of beneficial bacteria in 2022. At presentshe is the international sales director for the French biotech TargEDys - from Probiotics to PreciBiomics - the ambassador of precision probiotics, harnessing and translating science to products to bring the microbiome to the heart of healthcare. TargEDys is mostly known and recognized for *Hafnia alvei* HA4597, and its proven efficacy in weight management through the molecular mimicry of the hormone of satiety alpha-MSH by the bacteria metabolite ClpB.

Ashok K. Sharma

Ashok K. Sharma works as a postdoctoral scientist in Casero and Devkota Lab at the Inflammatory Bowel and Immunobiology Research Institute at Cedars Sinai Medical Center. The focus of his research is to identify probable mechanisms by which bacterial activities regulate immune responses in individuals who have been diagnosed with Ulcerative Colitis and Crohn's disease. He implements bioinformatics pipelines and machine-learning-based computational methods to analyse and integrate multi-omics datasets. Prior to this, he worked as a postdoctoral associate at the University of Minnesota- Twin Cities and was involved in the understanding of factors that impact gut microbial composition/function and its subsequent interactions with the host. Before starting his postdoctoral journey in the United States, he completed his bachelor's and master's in Pharmaceutical Sciences, followed by a PhD in Computational Biology from the Indian Institute of Science Education and Research in Bhopal, India.

He aims to keep applying AI/machine learning and other data-driven approaches to understand diet-microbiome-host interactions in animals and humans under diverse physiological conditions. Apart from this, he also intends to contribute to the areas of, microbiome-based diagnostics and therapeutics and personalized food and medicine to improve animal and human health using his expertise of data analysis skills.

Manuela Pausan

Manuela Pausan is a microbiome scientist who explores the interplay between the gut microbiome and herbal medicine to understand the roots of what makes a product microbiome-friendly. She is strongly interested in how the microbiome power can be harvested to improve health and prevent diseases, and which natural products can nourish the microbiome and keep it thriving. During her PhD tenure at the Medical University of Graz, she was involved in several microbiome-related projects which focused on the human archaeome and the importance of microbiome during pregnancy. She was awarded the L'Oréal Austria Fellowships for Women in Science in 2018. When she's not working on microbiome topics, she loves to enjoy exploring nature and also proactively uses her 'lab' skills to indulge in soap-making.

Alan Marsh

Alan completed his PhD with APC Microbiome Ireland, where he studied peptide antimicrobials and the microbial populations of fermented foods like kefir and kombucha. Following a break in his research to backpack across the world, Alan undertook a postdoc in microbiome research at the University of North Carolina Chapel Hill, where he is currently based. His work focuses on prebiotics, probiotics, and commensal gut populations.

Dr. Kristin Neumann

Dr. Kristin Neumann is the founder of the information platform 'MyMicrobiome' and a passionate scientist, with a PhD in Microbiology. Her professional career, through the scope of molecular biology and research on an antibiotic alternative led her to form 'MyMicrobiome'. Dr. Neumann's realization of the importance of an intact microbiome for an individual's physical well-being factored into her decision to summarize the science around the microbiome on the free information platform mymicrobiome.info.

The industry has already picked up on the microbiome trend and promises to improve the microbiome without regulation and very often without scientific evidence.

That is why 'MyMicrobiome' developed the world's first and only independent certification for microbiome-friendly cosmetics and personal care products (microbiome-friendly.com), one more step towards MyMicrobiome´s vision of a better, microbiome-friendly world.

Marco Pignatti

Marco Pignatti graduated in Medicine with 110 cum laude in 1995 from the University of Modena with a thesis titled 'Analysis of a computerized system for the multidimensional assessment of people with Down Syndrome' supervised by Prof. Claudio Franceschi. He specialized in Dermatology and Venereology in 2000 at the University of Modena.

He has worked in Prof. Carlo Pincelli's laboratory of cutaneous biology, dealing with the biology of keratinocytes with particular reference to the neurotrophins network and their receptors, apoptosis in the skin, skin stem cells, the effects of ultraviolet radiation on the skin, psoriasis and tumours skin, skin euro biology and neuro cosmetology. He has worked on the project 'THE ROLE OF SURVIVIN IN SKIN STEM CELLS' as part of the research group of Prof. Carlo Pincelli at the University of Modena and Reggio Emilia. He has also worked on the project: 'Molecular mechanisms underlying melanoma' of the research group under Prof. Carlo Pincelli, University of Modena and Reggio Emilia.

He developed a passion for the study of the relationships that link skin and its pathology with gut and its microbiota. In January 2017, he was given the first Dermobiotica Outpatient Clinic in a public facility within the Dermatological Clinic of the Policlinico of Modena.

He has written the books 'Dermobiotica. Alimentazione - Microbiota –Pelle'(Ed. Minerva Medica, 2018), ' Intestino e salute della pelle' (Terra Nuova, 2019), a children's book "I nostri piccoli amici' (Ed. YouCanPrint, 2020) and 'Manuale pratico di Dermobiotica' (Ed. Clorofilla, 2022).

Since 2017, he has been the President of the Italian Congress of Dermobiotica. He also speaks at numerous conferences, courses and webinars on the role of the microbiota in dermatology. He gave a talk titled 'The gut-microbiota-skin axis' at the World Congress of Dermatology, WCD 2019.

Sofia Popov

Sofia Popov is the founder of GUTXY ("gut-see") the first consumer microbiome testing company in Denmark. Her work at GUTXY focuses on running dietary interventions that compare how different dietary habits affect the abundance of various species in the gut, and how this can impact digestion and improve overall gut wellness. Her background lies in Biological Sciences (BSc) and Bioinformatics (MSc.) During her masters at the University of Copenhagen, her thesis investigated the role different dietary fibres play on the gut composition. Sofia is passionate about communicating the different aspects of microbiome science and making it more accessible, allowing everyone to make health-conscious and sustainable lifestyle choices keeping their gut microbes in mind.

ABOUT THE LETSAUTHOR COMMUNITY

At LetsAuthor, we are building a community of experts and professionals to come together and write books on a variety of topics. We believe that each one of us has a unique story to tell, an experience to share, and we are giving you the opportunity to be heard, to make a difference. We follow the philosophy of Open Authoring. We open each of our books to everyone who wants to participate. We choose the contributions that are most valuable to our readers, carefully validate the content, weave a beautiful story that our readers will love, and present a brand-new book to the world, one at a time! If you too have a story or an experience to share and would like to become a part of our author community, please visit https:// letsauthor.com/ and sign up as a Lead Author or a Contributor. Please let us know the areas you would like to contribute, and we will consider opening a new book if one isn't already in the making.

https://letsauthor.com/

OUR EARLY BACKERS

A BIG THANK YOU to our early backers, who believed enough in
I, Microbiome and LetsAuthor to pre-order a copy, when it was merely
a landing page.

– Co-Authors, *I, Microbiome*

Kumar Sankaran

Rachel Jessey

Gaurang Ramesh

Jakov Minic

Paul Denny-Gouldson

Beatrix Förster

Luis E F Dantas

Novak Rogic

Dragana Nikolic

Radouane Oudrhiri

Dusan Cucak

Chris Georgiou

Dr Biljana Simonovikj

Lucía Diez Gutiérrez

Ricardo Carvalho

Rwivoo Baruah

Ujjwala Bhati

Ivana Filipovic Yorke

Alexander
Sulakvelidze

Simone Giesler

Duda Markovic

Jürgen Gross

Barbara Janssens

Ahmed Hashmi

Milka Sokolovic

Ferencz Sandor Paldy

Dr. Darja Wagner

Dusica Rados

Natasa
Moravic-Balkanski

Sagar Aryal

Valentine Favrod

Sanja Mihajlovic

Ana Perovic

Jack Alexander

Tina Quinn

Draginja Kovacevic

Sanja Matic

Tatjana Turner

Timo Spring

Vera Troselj

Gabriele Malengo

Selma Lazovic

Danka Vuga

Helena Otašević

Yuki Oguchi

Thorsten Umland

Sergio Manzano
Gomez

Jelena Anacker

Deeksha Garg

Abhinav Dey

Sushant Kumar

Viswanadham D

Ragini Rai

Pariksha Rao

Ashok Gopinath

Sanjiv Kumar

Jiri Snaidr

Debojit Guha

Sneha Murthy

Romi Gupta

Vineeth Vasu

Sankar Bhattacharyya

Beena Pillai

Tanja Ninkovic

Samriddha Ray

Hamsa Bhargavi

Dana Buckman

Christian Dieckmann

Rod Dickerson

John Burton

Gerald Dard

Sebastian Wahl

Larry Weiss

Christiane Gras

Catherine Rhodes

Johan Wahlqvist

Felix Faupel

Nicole Liammari

Sathya Janardhanan

Diana Høtoft

Kelly Eden

Ashley Tucker

Verena Suchanek Champié

Lorenzo Miorelli

Dorian Delclos

Adela Eller

Roger Frechette

Zhi Yang Loh

Sheryl Tan

Brendan Burns

Leanne Levy

Ewa Hudson

Sangeeta Choudhury

John Wilson

Gregory Bonfilio

Sharath Chandra Arandkar

Sven Sewitz

Vikas Pandey

Sara De Monte

Diane Lince

Vera A Ortiz

Mina Nicoletti

Cicely Washington

Irene Predazzi

Phan Nguyen

Geoffrey Hamilton

Cynthia Lawley

Ludovic Meilhac

Swati Kadam

Marc Philouze

Jonathan Dornell

Harry Glorikian

Susan Knowles

Téo Fournier

Tyler Morris

Seema Patel

Clotilde teiling

Sommer Erik

Abhishek Mohanty

Dr. Sanjay Nipanikar

Bhagat Singh Rajput

Naveen Chava

Anthony Finbow

Jack Alexander

Sagar Ramteke

Kylene Guse

Siddarth Selvaraj

Narendra Malhotra

Sanjay Sachdeva

John McNamara

Ericka Ramko

Santosh Kuruvilla

Kiirsten Suurkask

Emmanuelle Costard

Blair Holbrook

Shikha Obrien

Usman Qazi

Paul Bromann

Asim Bikas Das

Malathy Krishnamurthy

Venkat Subramani

Arjun Srinivasan

Andreas Dietzel

Meena Kalyanaraman

Sunita Parasuraman

Lata Sundaram

Usha Sankar

Vijay Mani

Massimo Barberi

Jean-Christophe Gadrat

Annachiara De Prisco

Ajitha Rajan

Ashwini Sankar

Venkatraman Arakoni

Pradeep Venkatachalam

Sarat C Sekar

Shwetha Mangalesh

Abhijeet
Dharmapurikar
Dilip Chabria
Radha Raman Pandey
Sandeep Kunkunuru
Balaji Iyer
Poornima Srinivasan
Punith Raj KN
Dr Gargi Roy
Goswami
Lincoln Jacob
Vivek Bharadwaj
Vishwanath
Venkatachalam
Suniti sundaram
Amar Kar
Csorba Cintia
Debjani Saha
Inge Lindseth
Krishna Pantakani
Becky Upton
Marco Pane
Simona Ardemagni
Marco Pignatti
PH Richardson
Emilie Maret
Deben Dey
Ionut Birlad
Umberto Argese
Shabnam Kar
Suman Kapoor
Murugan Subramanian
Elvira Gammarota
Paolo Magnolfi
Paolo Magnolfi

Matthew Dougherty
Adrian Kladnig
Norbert Bomba
Jana Racková
Michael Tippie
Francisco de Abreu e
Lima
Heiner Oberkampf
Felipe Perez
Christopher Likins
Kate Marie Forbes
Vi Van Phan
Tara Gupta
Cerezo, Silvia
Tiss Méheut
Kevin Burdin
Timo Werneke
Michelle McDonald
George Alb
Vivekanandan
Muthukrishnan
Barbara Putz
Ana Cvetkovic
Shelly Ann Winokur
Geoffry Smith
Oliver Hvarre
Supriya Bidanta
Tanja Walbrunn
Josefine Hiller Pongo
Krista Parry
Louise Deering
Sophia Hasselt
Benedetta Mannini
Twiggy Hedwig Scheck
Sarah de Visser

Michael Chou
Miriam Bittel
Christoph Strehl
Len Monheit
Laura Frazier
Petra Nikell
Daniel Kammerer
Anna Soine
Teresa Petraia
Paul Hammer
Sophie Stephens
Anita Golani
Günter Schneider
Nova Morgan
Beatrice Ranieri
Maria Zimmermann
Gesa Richter
Sandra Santos
Laura Lodi
Louise Thomas-Minns
Beatrice Venturi
Catanzaro
Claire Vink
Wauter Delvaux
LS Ramdin
Luisa Di Luzio
Roxane Bakker
Irina Mircea
Thomas Demuyser
Christine Vigne-Bimai
Eva Schirmeier
Mariarosaria Matera
nishchitha jagadeesh
Ilaria Cavecchia
Amarti